Put Old on Hold

Put Old on Hold

Barbara Morris

Image F/X Publications
Escondido, California

Put Old on Hold by Barbara Morris, R.Ph.

Image F/X Publications, P.O. Box 937, Escondido, CA 92033-0937
Phone: 760-480-2710; Fax: 760-480-9959
Website: www.putoldonhold.com

DISCLAIMER: This publication is designed to provide accurate and authoritative information with regard to the subject matter covered. It is sold with the understanding that the publisher is not engaged in rendering legal, medical, or other professional services. If medical advice or other expert health care assistance is required, the services of a competent professional should be sought.

Cover design by
Text design and layout by Robert Goodman, Silvercat™, San Diego, California

0 9 8 7 6 5 4 3 2 1

Cataloging in Publication Data

Morris, Barbara.

Put old on hold / Barbara Morris. -- Escondido, CA :
Image F/X Publications, 2004

p. / cm.
ISBN: 0-9667842-2-7

1. Longevity. 2. Aging--Prevention.
3. Longetivity--Nutritional aspects. 4. Health.
I. Title.

RA776.75 .M67 2004
612.6/8--dc22 CIP

Printed in the United States of America

To my husband, Marty

for his love, constant encouragement, unfailing good humor, positive outlook and, above of all, for always remembering that I am a goddess and treating me as such. And he never fails to let me know when my tiara is askew.

Contents

Acknowledgements xi

Foreword by Brandon Barnum xiii

Why I Wrote This Book 3

I'm Telling it Like It Is: The Truth about Aging . . . 7

The Origins of Oldness 9

The Three Basics of Agelessness 13

Health 14

Retirement 14

Attitude 14

Health 15

Nothing Matters More 15

A Personal Responsibility 17

No Butts about It 19

Be Aggressive about Your Health 22

The Importance of Lifestyle 27

Health Care Realities 29

The State of Health Care Today 29

Health Care Rationing 33

Free Yourself from Fear of the Future 34
Educate Yourself! 37
Partner with Your Practitioner 39
Too Much of a Good Thing 40
Stamp Out Food Abuse 45
The Classic Signs of Food Abuse 46
Why We Abuse Food 47
The Supermarket: Temple of Temptations 48
Miles of Not So Incredible Edibles 51
Buy Now, Pay Later 53
Supplements and Why We Need Them 54
Supplementation Is a Personal Choice 56
What Your Doctor or Pharmacist
May Not Tell You 56
The Anti-Aging Supplements:
Your Secret Weapon 58
Additional Information on Supplements 61
Other Possible Supplements 62
Water, Water Everywhere, But Who Stops to Drink? . . 64
How Much Water is Enough? 65
The Wonders of Water Consumption 68
Can Water Hold a Cure? 70
What Every Consumer Needs
to Know About Medications 72
Problems with Multiple Medications 75
The CBC Power Packed Profile 76
Insider Information: Be in the Know 79

Retirement 83
We Need a New Perspective 83
Why Retire? 85
Retirement Realities 89
Retirement Reality No. 1:
Loss of Income and Decline in Quality of Life . . . 90
Retirement Reality No. 2:
Difficulty Going Back to Work 93
Retirement Reality No. 3:
Loss of Self Esteem and Personal Power 94
Retirement Reality No. 4:
Adopting the Senior Lifestyle 98
Retirement Reality No. 5:
Unproductive Use of Time 100
Alternative to Retirement: Seamless Living 104
Your Bolt of Life 105
Preparing for Your Second Life 107
Attitude **111**
Agelessness Begins with Attitude 111
Avoid Limitation Thinking 114
Appreciate and Associate with Younger People . . 117
Trust Your Ability 119
Twenty Rules to Get it All Together 121
Exercise! 121
Observe Others 126
Constantly Look for Inspiring Role Models 126
Be a Positive Role Model Yourself 130
Maintain an Inventory of Your Skills 131
Defy Convention: Be a Rebel with a Cause 132

Cultivate a Sense of Humor and
a Realistic Perspective 134
Be Kind and Patient 135
Wear a Pleasant Expression 136
Don't Play Age Games 137
Say You Feel Terrific 137
Keep Your Appearance Contemporary 138
Consider Medical and Dental Enhancement 141
Watch Your Posture 144
Visualize Your Future 145
Just Say No to the Deadly Sins
of Negative Self Talk 149
Do Not Worship in The Church
of Chronological Age 159
Be a Birthday Party Pooper 164
Better than a Party:
The Blast That Lasts All Year 167
Gods and Goddesses Just do it! 170
Mission Possible: Putting Old on Hold 171
The Opportunity of a Lifetime 180
Resources 183
Index 187
Barbara Morris' Personal Anti-Aging Program . . 195
About the Author 201

Acknowledgements

Writing a book is a team effort that requires the talent of many people. I've been extremely fortunate to have the help of some of the best, and here they are:

Antoinette Kuritz, my incredible publicist. Every author wants a great publicist; very few are fortunate enough to find one. I'm one of the fortunate few. Antoinette is assisted by her two talented children, Jared, also a publicist, and Alyscia, an editor. The fresh innovative thinking and youthful enthusiasm of this dynamic trio is incredible. How did I get so lucky?

Leslie Charles, my amazing content editor. There are not enough superlatives to adequately express my gratitude for her editing skills and the countless ways she has helped me.

Robert Goodman, my award-winning master designer who produced the book interior and helped with important details.

Gerry Williams, my patient and extraordinary photographer who did the cover photos.

Michael Lynch, my cover designer who cheerfully endured countless requests for changes.

Kathleen Strattan, my meticulous indexer — an absolute joy to work with.

In addition to the above extraordinary people, I am grateful to everyone who contributed to this book, including but not limited to:

Actress Florence Henderson, an incredibly gracious woman who gave advice and encouragement;

Brandon Barnum, CEO of Longevity Labs, who has encouraged and supported my mission of healthy agelessness;

Psychologist Dr. Victor Kops, for confirming my belief that healthy agelessness can and should become the norm.

Foreword by Brandon Barnum

Take Action to Challenge the Aging Process

Over the past decade, medical scientists have made tremendous advancements in the field of anti-aging medicine. From the decoding of the human genome to the use of pluripotent stem cells for tissue and organ regeneration, scientists are discovering how to control the biological aging process on a cellular level.

Over the next twenty years, these advancements will radically change the face of medicine and dramatically improve quality of life for aging Americans. Yet despite these scientific advancements, the most important factor in human longevity continues to be a healthy lifestyle. While we once assumed heredity was the dominating force in how we age, how we choose to live from day to day is the key.

The benefits of a healthy lifestyle are well documented and well publicized. Yet, despite all of the information on diet and exercise, over 30 percent of all Americans are considered clinically obese. That's a frightening statistic when you consider that obesity contributes to three of the leading causes of death in the United States: heart disease (31.4 percent), cancer (23.3 percent), and stroke (6.9 percent)

The decisions you make on a daily basis directly affect your body's physiological rate of aging. Your dietary habits, exercise routines, stress management capabilities, and attitude will either cause your body to become weak and feeble, or help your body retain a vital, energetic, and youthful version of your current self.

Understand that lack of action *is* an action. If you are serious about maximizing your longevity and physical quality of life, you must start taking positive steps to keep your brain, vital organs, and tissues nourished while simultaneously strengthening your muscles, joints, and bones. A great place to start is by adopting the techniques outlined in this book, *Put Old on Hold.*

Put Old on Hold is the best anti-aging book available. Unlike most books on this topic, this one is written with the average reader in mind, outlining a program that is extremely easy to follow. Barbara's experience as a pharmacist has taught her how to transfer professional counseling into book form. In reading this book I often felt as if I was standing at the pharmacy window being advised by my local expert.

The single most important point Barbara makes is taking personal responsibility for your health. Regardless of how wonderful your health care providers are, you are ultimately responsible for the well being of every cell in your body. If you nourish and protect your cells, they will serve you well. If you deprive or abuse them, they will degenerate and decay. It's your choice.

Barbara knows that no generation grasps this reality better than Baby Boomers. In watching their parents and grandparents struggle with debilitating diseases such as cancer, diabetes, and Alzheimer's disease, a high percentage of Boomers are taking a proactive approach to health and wellness.

Today, Boomers represent 28 percent of the U.S. population. At 76 million strong, they represent the largest single sustained population surge in the history of the United States. The massive wealth, power and influence controlled by this generation give them the ability to drive changes in modern medicine. This generation understands that the body, mind, and spirit all play a role in health and wellness; its members demand that physicians diagnose and treat them holistically, rather than as a sum of their parts.

Over the next two decades, you will witness Boomers igniting a revolution in the medical field. Integrative wellness will become the norm. Health care will become extremely proactive, incorporating cellular diagnostic techniques to monitor cellular changes throughout your lifetime. Modern western medicine will be combined with Eastern philosophies to treat your entire being. Customized nutritional supplementation will emerge to provide your body with the precise formulation of nutrients needed for your individual biochemistry.

We are a nation that is food rich but nutrition poor. Thousands of clinical studies have shown that today's most common diseases are caused by the lack of proper nutrient intake.

Scientists have shown that supplementing your diet with essential vitamins, minerals, herbs, and hormones can help you maintain a youthful physiology and prevent most illnesses from developing. By giving your body the optimal level of important nutrients, you can reduce symptoms and dramatically improve your overall health. Clearly, when it comes to longevity, healthy nutritional habits are essential.

In countries such as Japan, where diet consists mainly of whole foods, unprocessed and low in fat, records consistently show low rates of obesity, heart disease, osteoporosis, memory loss, and breast, colon, or prostate cancer. Typically the people in these cultures are physically younger than their chronological ages, proof positive that adopting healthy lifestyle habits can dramatically improve longevity.

Of course, the primary objective in anti-aging medicine is not just to extend a person's lifespan, but to increase the number of active, healthy, and vital years lived. As president of Longevity Labs, my focus is on improving each client's entire quality of life. Our goal is to help people enjoy their senior years with the same physical abilities and function as people in their thirties and forties.

Over the years, I have read countless books from self-proclaimed anti-aging experts. *Put Old on Hold* truly is the first book that provides a straightforward program for stopping the physical and mental signs of aging, with strategies proven to keep both mind and body feeling young and vital.

Barbara Morris proves that the aging process can be controlled, radiating more vitality and energy than women two decades younger. She is truly a shining example that the aging process can be controlled by maintaining a healthy life-style, regular activity, and a youthful attitude.

I personally challenge you to adopt the easy-to-follow lifestyle techniques outlined in this book. Making these simple changes in diet, exercise, stress relief, and nutritional supplementation can add years to your life and life to your years.

Brandon Barnum
President and CEO, Longevity Labs Inc.
www.LongevityLabs.net

Foreword by Victor Kops

If you want to live a healthier and a longer life, Barbara Morris' *Put Old On Hold* is for you. The sooner one adopts a healthier lifestyle, the better. And *Put Old On Hold* provides practical advice to do just that.

A practicing pharmacist for more than 30 years, the author is used to giving concrete advice on a daily basis. Her tell-it-like-it-is style makes the book eminently readable. And to her credit, there is no scientific/medical babble in this book. However, neither is it a theoretical discussion. The author, at 74, still works full-time and looks far younger than her years. Her energy level is a living testimony to her lifestyle choices. Barbara's advice has certainly worked for her, and there is no good reason why it cannot help you.

Living a healthy life is a matter of choice. While genetics do play a part, they usually only account for about one-third of physical illnesses. The rest is up to us.

It has long been widely accepted that if people eat properly, get a good night's rest, do not overwork, exercise regularly, avoid stress, do not drink excessively, and do not smoke, they will probably maintain good health. Treating your mind and body properly increases the probability that you will live a fuller and longer life. It is a prescription that we all need to consider. But, according to Morris, there is more.

The aging process can certainly be slowed, and habit and lifestyle do contribute. For example, it is widely known that smoking produces premature wrinkling and, worse yet, it can be fatal. As Morris rightfully points out, nicotine addiction is the most reversible health problem in America. Cigarettes kill approximately 400,000 Americans per year. Ironically, hard drugs such as heroin and cocaine kill less than 50,000 people per year. For every cigarette smoked, the average person will live eight minutes less. Consider that fate before you light up! But, as Morris suggests, you must also consider eating habits, exercise, and stress reduction as part of your anti-aging regime.

It is most refreshing that as a pharmacist, the author does not push medication. She does, however, encourage her reader to select a physician with whom he or she can partner. Her advice is to seek out a doctor who is interested in you as a whole person and not just a collection of symptoms needed to be dispensed with in seven-minute intervals. And she points out that finding a knowledgeable and caring pharmacist is also important.

Emphasizing the proposition that we should not expect a pill to cure our poor choices, Morris suggests that before we medicate, we assess what lifestyle modifications would alleviate our symptoms.

As a psychologist, Morris' focus on personal responsibility for overall health and the aging process intrigued me. Placing the responsibility for our health on health-care professionals is easy; it passes the buck. But for Morris, the buck stops with the individual. Encouraging each of us to make the most of our health, to employ powerful anti-aging strategies, and to take responsibility for the attitude with which we handle the aging process is empowering.

Morris' information on vitamins and supplements alone is worth the price of this book. In the past decade, there has been an explosion of information and misinformation on what we should be ingesting on a daily basis. This knowledgeable pharmacist separates fact from fiction in words that we can all understand. With no vested interest in selling any of these products, her objectivity is a welcome relief.

Whether you are in your 20's and just starting your adult journey, or in your 50's and facing senior status, Morris's practical, informative, responsible approach to health and anti-aging will be of physical and emotional benefit to you. Aging is a part of life, and Morris does not deny this. But it is the manner in which we age, and the quality of life we can and should expect, that are of concern in her book. Morris' strategies make sense. Her advice is practical and easy to implement. All it takes is the right attitude, the right mindset. With the mind/body connection already firmly established, Morris' advice is a powerful, essential tool in the quest for continuing health.

Victor Kops, Ph.D.
Licensed Psychologist
Fellow, San Diego Psychological Association

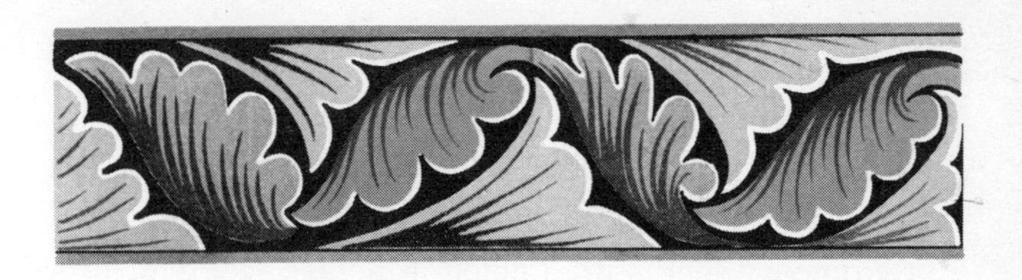

Why I Wrote This Book

I wrote *Put Old on Hold* for those who want to enjoy a long, healthy, and productive life, and want help to reach that goal. I know that while preserving the attributes of youth is a challenge, maintaining youthful physical and mental characteristics is definitely doable today.

Old age is a state of mind as well as a culturally assigned chronological number. Not too long ago, "old" was age 65, and then age eighty-five. Currently our country has more centenarians than ever. But reaching the 100 mark is no longer a reliable indicator of old age. In an average month in 1999, 50,000 people age 90 and above were in the workforce. In a society that views old people as incapable of being as productive as young workers are, this is worth noting. Indeed, the concept of old age is changing and improving rapidly, and in ways never dreamed possible, even as recent as 25 years ago.

Two distinct models for aging exist in our society: The dominant traditional "senior culture," which involves a state of mind and way of living that invites decline and dependence;

and the new, growing "ageless culture" consisting of innovative ways and techniques to put old on hold. The latter adheres to a new way of being that defies decline and dependence while promoting healthy, productive, ageless longevity.

Gerontology gurus are finding it increasingly difficult to clarify when what we call old age actually occurs, or even what it is. Their search for a definition is difficult because it is not a disease, a number, or a condition. It's a choice. To a great extent, a healthy individual can control mental and physical elements of old age by staying aware of personal changes, practicing an aggressive maintenance regimen, and refusing to allow age-related decline to gain a toehold.

I believe it's possible to put old on hold indefinitely. I'm doing it; I've discovered some "Super Keys" to healthy agelessness and I share them in this book. My perspective is not for contented, traditional retirees. I wouldn't want or attempt to disturb their bliss. This book is for those who wish to live in a state of seamless, evolutionary productive growth, with youthful élan for as long as they live, which should be for a very long time. In the past century, the American lifespan has increased a phenomenal 27 years so there is a lot more time to enjoy an unprecedented "second life." I challenge you to have the vision, imagination and commitment to go for it!

I'm now 74 years of age, not 74 years old. Normally, I do not reveal my age, and in this youth worshipping culture I suggest you don't either. Your age is as personal as your bank balance, and you wouldn't reveal your financial worth to just anyone. By declining to reveal your age, you live with greater freedom, avoiding some of the limitations our culture places on age numbers.

For example, if you appear younger than you are, you will not likely hear depressing comments or questions such as "You are too old to do that," or "Why are you still working at your age?" If ever asked the latter question and you are a woman, your answer should be that you have child support and alimony payments to make. Then wait for the reaction. It's fun.

The only reason I'm disclosing my age is so you can appreciate that I know what I'm talking about. I'm sure you'd prefer to learn how to put old on hold from someone who is actually living her message rather than from a forty-something "expert" who has poured over scientific journals and interviewed a multitude of old folks, pretending that he or she has all the answers. In this case, experience beats theory!

My take on chronological age is this: Age is an accounting of time gone by. It's a useful identifier for certain legal purposes but our culture goes far beyond that, attaching undue importance to "the numbers." We specify parameters of behavior and expected standards of being for each decade, thereby assigning how much or how little people should be getting out of life. Rebels who live outside of the boundaries of acceptable behavior for a given chronological age often have a hard row to hoe. Admonitions to "act your age" can shoot down achievable aspirations that could potentially change the world. What a loss!

Chronological age has little relationship to ability or state of health. I believe it is far more important to focus on biological or physiological age: How well the mind/body connection functions and maintains itself. Biological age is the age that really matters and, I promise, you have enormous control over it. You *can* put old on hold and you can begin today.

I am so excited about my discoveries on how to achieve healthy agelessness and I want to share what I know with you. When I meet someone younger than I who is not aging well, I want to grab and shake the person and scream, "Hey! You are aging prematurely! It doesn't have to be that way. Listen to me . . . I can help you stop old age in its tracks." Well, accosting a stranger with that kind of rhetoric would likely go over like a lead balloon. But you are reading this book because you chose to, so you and I are not strangers – we are friends. And as friends will, they sometimes "exchange words" because they care! Therefore, I will be doing a lot of preaching at you, my friend, and you are entitled to preach back, and that's okay. Thanks for coming along for the journey through these pages. I know you will be glad you did, and I hope that at the conclusion you will write to me when and let me know how I helped or motivated you to put old on hold.

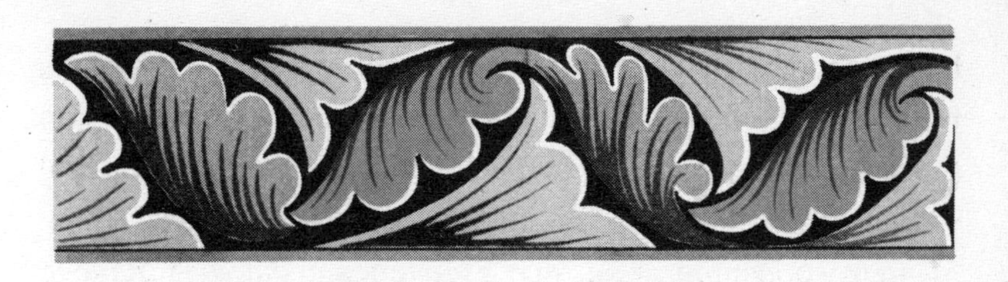

I'm Telling It Like It Is: The Truth about Aging

Some of my friends accuse me of being preachy, like a geriatric Judge Judy. Such an appraisal offends me greatly because, as you can tell, I am more positive and more charming than Her Honor. On the other hand, maybe you can't tell just yet. But stay with me – I am both charming and disarming, especially when I preach.

Here's my excuse for preaching, if and when I do. Telling people what to do is a way of life for me. I'm a pharmacist and people ask all kinds of questions such as, "What can I take for my backache?" or "I've got this hacking cough that keeps me up all night. What will make it go away?" or "Hey, does that stuff they advertise to perk up your love life really work and which one works best?" (For the record, I don't know of any that work!) No kidding, people assume I'm an expert and that I have a solution for every ailment or problem a human can experience. Since I'm not a physician nor licensed to practice medicine, I usually offer several appropriate suggestions, preach if I think it will help, and then leave the final decision to the customer.

I unabashedly admit to "telling it like it is" when it comes to aging. Far too many of us get old too fast and it doesn't have to happen. Every fiber of my being believes that the various types and levels of decline typically seen with advancing age are not inevitable. In spite of what seems to be irrefutable evidence, in spite of so-called expert knowledge in the field of aging – in spite of it all – I maintain that you can control both the quality and progression of the aging process. But you may ask, how can I say that in the face of what appears normal or obvious? Just look at the elderly people around in various stages of decline. How can I make such an assertion? It's easy. It has become clear to me that much of the physical and mental decline traditionally associated with the aging process is nothing more than the result of a lifetime of abuse (food, tobacco, alcohol), mental mismanagement (negative, defeatist thinking), and neglect (failure to take care of what you have).

There always have been certain "truths" known to us resulting from observation, assumption, tradition, and pronouncements of so-called experts. But are irrefutable truths always true? Here are some "truths" now recognized as false:

The earth is flat. If you get to close to the edge, you will surely fall off.

Crops fail and animals die because of spells cast by evil witches. Burn the witches and all will be well.

A high fever indicates too much blood in the body. To cure the patient, apply leeches to the body to suck out excess blood.

At one time each of the above so-called truths was the result of the understanding, knowledge, and prejudices of the era in which they existed. To have disregarded or spoken against them was heretical. Yet, it has since been proven the earth is not flat, crop failures and plagues are not the result of evil spells, and the blood letting practiced during the Middle Ages is quackery.

Countless untouchable truths once held as gospel now reside in the realm of the ridiculous. Many so-called truths carved in stone of our time relating to aging now deserve the same fate. When it comes to getting older many of us tenaciously cling to "the earth is flat" mentality, meaning we accept it without argument. It's a given that people *will* suffer mental and physical decline with passing years, but it can be abated, managed and controlled far more than we think. As you read this book you'll become aware of many detrimental contemporary "truths", while discovering how you can avoid and overcome their negative effect on your health, happiness, and longevity.

The Origins of Oldness

Let me offer some new truths about aging, while addressing some of the outdated ideas responsible for the condition we recognize as oldness. I defy anyone to prove any of the following are wrong:

Oldness results from a lack of understanding of, and failure to embrace what constitutes an anti-aging diet and lifestyle. It results from an unclear understanding of why we age at all and how we can stave off the process. Two anti-aging theories that make the most sense to me are the Free Radical Theory of aging, and the restricted calorie, but highly nutritious diet.

To put it simply, the Free Radical Theory of aging holds that the process of living, (eating, breathing, metabolic breakdown, exposure to environmental stresses, and the buildup of toxins) results in the formation of reactive "free radicals" — very unstable molecules that attack DNA and healthy cells, stealing electrons to achieve stability. This "raiding" of healthy cells eventually results in cellular death and thus, signs of aging. What is exciting and promising is that free radicals are controllable with diet and supplements called anti-oxidants.

The restricted calorie theory of aging has been around since the 1930s and it has gained increased legitimacy as more anti-aging researchers focus their work on it. They conclude that a restricted calorie theory is extremely promising as a tool to control aging. The key is not just calorie reduction – the diet also has to be highly nutritious and tasty, which is a difficult combination to achieve.

What we think of as oldness results largely from plain laziness; you know what you should or could do to help yourself, but maintenance and prevention feel like too much work. By willful neglect, you set yourself up to become a victim, if not now, then in the future. When joints begin to creak or feel painful; when cholesterol and high blood pressure shoot out of sight; when you develop diabetes – you blame God, the government, your doctor, the weather, and uncaring friends or family for your compromised physical condition. I recall a woman whose bone density test showed she had osteopenia (early osteoporosis). Her doctor made several recommendations to improve her condition, including weight-bearing exercises. She laughed at that suggestion, saying, "That's not going to happen." When I asked why not, she wailed, "I'm too lazy to exercise!" So much for the "it's in the genes" or "old age just happens to everyone" excuses.

Oldness occurs because we are unaware of the forces of gradualism and how we are changing over time. Youth is deceptive. It makes us arrogant. The seemingly unchanged image we see in the mirror each day is slowly and gradually slipping away. Although we look we don't really see the small steady changes. The subtle changes we fail to see keep most of us from engaging in aggressive maintenance and prevention. After all, when we hope and believe we will be young forever, that the gift of youth will remain ours with little or no input from us, we have little incentive to do what is necessary to maintain what we have. We look at stooped, unsteady old people and believe we will never get to that place or condition. That's what I mean by arrogance, and that's what youth and lack of awareness will do if we allow it.

Oldness results from unquestioned, uncritical observation. We see peers aging and how family members or friends have aged. We assume the outcomes are inevitable, so we do nothing to stop or reverse the decline. *Everybody gets old. That's the way it is.* Not only do we make assumptions and let things happen; we unintentionally copy thinking and behaviors: "Monkey see, monkey do."

Oldness results from expectation. This is where the "earth is flat" mentality really kicks in. Regardless of what we do, we "know" we will get old and decrepit, so why fight it? After all, that's one of those irrefutable truths. We forget another old maxim that holds more than a grain of truth: *You basically get what you expect in life.*

Oldness results from retirement. Once we internalize the concept called retirement, (which the subconscious interprets as a time of preparation for death) the mind and body begin to shut down in anticipation of the final event. Denial, staying busy, or distracting ourselves doesn't slow or impede the process because the mind has accepted the finality of the decision to retire. The human mind and body cannot lie fallow and fare well. We must grow or die!

I encourage you to think about what oldness means to you, how you perceive it, at what age you think it occurs, and how you will face it: With resignation or revitalization.

The Three Basics of Agelessness

This book covers three basic subjects necessary to put old on hold:

- Health
- Retirement
- Attitude

If you understand and adopt the essence of these powerful concepts into your thinking and behavior you can easily put old on hold. If you do, you will experience an incredible, enviable second life after age 60; a precious gift too few people possess. At a time when conventional wisdom says you should be in a state of decline, you will be the youthful exception. Unbelievers will dismiss you as one of the fortunate few born with good genes. So choose to be exceptional. When you work at it, a good genetic package becomes a great one. Believe it will happen, act on it, and agelessness will be yours!

Health

The condition of your health and your ability to maintain it in an optimum state, plus your determination to constantly improve it will affect your ability to put old on hold. Nothing is more important.

Retirement

When you retire or how you retire plays an important role in your ability to put old on hold. If at traditional retirement age you change jobs or do what you've always wanted to do that's productive and challenging, that's not retirement. It's only retirement when you allow your mind and body to turn to mush.

Attitude

Having an independent, tough "march to your own drummer" mindset about aging and using the right tools to develop agelessness will determine how youthfully you age. Be willing to thumb your nose at conventional wisdom and outdated myths or mentality about aging. Gladly suffer the envy of those who are in a state of decline and would like to drag you down with them, while being a source of inspiration and encouragement for those trying to avoid decline. Invite them to join you in your quest for agelessness. By helping others, you ultimately help yourself.

Health

Nothing Matters More

Good health is your most important asset and prized possession. Acquiring and maintaining it must be a consuming priority. Your health is more important than money, sex, power, possessions or relationships. With great health, money is not a worry, sex is better, power is awesome, possessions are a pleasure, and relationships are what you choose to make them. Optimum health provides liberation beyond measure. It is so freeing that it boggles the imagination. Excellent physical and mental health will enable you to revel in life over seventy. I guarantee it.

At a healthy age 60, you can be much smarter and wiser than in your younger years. You finally understand what's important and what's not. Liberated from youthful concerns, you are free to do what you've always wanted to do. When I say you can have a second life, that's exactly what I mean. It's an unprecedented gift to enjoy if you play your cards right early enough in the game. In your second life, you won't have to muddle through the terrible teenage years and suffer through a mid-life crisis all over again. The youthful struggles of "getting there" will be gone. You will "be there" and you can use your valuable past life experience to grow on. Your second life will epitomize the essence of Martin Luther King Jr.'s proclamation, "Free at Last! Free at Last!"

Yes, the essence of putting old on hold is freedom, opportunity, and choice! You can go back to school, begin a new career, start a new business, enjoy a new relationship, or whatever. You can have a job that provides a great standard of living rather than just getting by on Social Security. If you are in good health and have adequate income, you can enjoy some of the finer things in life rather than having to spend your money on medication, and cheap, low nutrition foods.

Putting old on hold is about freedom from fear. When you are healthy and strong, you don't have to worry about being a victim of mental, physical, or financial abuse, or fall prey to social systems that limit your freedom or security. The best part about putting old on hold may be the freedom you give to your children. When you are 60, 70, and beyond, and in great health, your Boomer-age children, with inevitable problems of their own, won't have to worry, "Will we have to put Mom and Dad in a nursing home?" or "Will they have to (God forbid) come and live with us in our place?" or "Will we have to help them pay their medical expenses?"

The benefits of putting old on hold are too great to pass up. Do it for yourself, do it for your kids, and do it for society. One less ailing, dependent person needing public assistance is a kindness to your taxpaying neighbors. We all benefit from each other's great health.

Don't fret; putting old on hold is not a grueling process or unrelenting work. It's an exciting challenge and an opportunity to do what you want to do with your life, regardless of chronological age. It's being able at 60, 70 and beyond, to look great, feel like a kid, be productive, anticipate the future and say, "Wow! This is amazing! Why hasn't everyone figured this out?" Because you are reading this, consider yourself one of the lucky ones who will learn to apply the secrets of agelessness. I know the way intimately, so stay with me!

A Personal Responsibility

I urge you to never lose sight of the truth that your health is your most precious possession. I'll remind you of that repeatedly because internalizing health consciousness is a preface to everything you think and do. Adjust your attitude until you can joyfully embrace your health as your first and foremost concern.

Here's the first step in taking responsibility for your health. Recognize that your health and your well-being are in your hands. This should be a given, but not everyone realizes the extent to which this is true. So I'll clarify: It's not your spouse's responsibility, your parents' responsibility, your children's responsibility, the government's responsibility, or your doctor's responsibility. Your health maintenance is *your* responsibility.

One day, as a woman picked up prescriptions for high blood pressure and cholesterol, she asked if I could also ring up a couple of romance novels. Each book was about two inches thick, so it appeared she spent a lot of time reading. When I asked this woman if she took as much time reading about her medical problems, she replied, "Oh, that's my doctor's responsibility. He's being paid to worry about it."

Wrong answer! Her doctor may be a very caring person, but should she expect her physician to worry about her health? I don't think so. There are limits to a doctor's responsibility. Treatment, yes. Worry, no. When doctors leave the office at night, they're like everybody else. They have worries and concerns of their own. Your health habits are under your personal jurisdiction!

In contrast, when another customer came in to pick up a prescription for her high cholesterol, even before she paid for it, she asked about side effects. In doing her research she discovered that the medication the doctor had prescribed was potentially harmful to the liver. She asked me to comment on her findings.

Rather than tell her my opinion, I showed her the comprehensive information sheet manufacturers are required to provide with every package of medication. It includes all of the known potential side effects. Let me suggest that when you have a prescription filled, always ask the pharmacist for the "package insert." You probably won't understand 90 percent of what it says, but you will understand the description of side effects.

After reading the list of possible side effects, which indeed did include the possibility of liver damage, she said, "Never mind. I won't take the medication if it's okay with you. I've lowered my cholesterol before with diet and I can do it again. It won't be fun, but at least I'll have a healthy liver."

That's what I mean by taking responsibility. You may be wondering what might happen if she is unable to lower her cholesterol to an acceptable level this time. Common sense says she may opt for the medication. But first, she will improve her diet and take full responsibility for the results. This woman certainly has the ability to have a fabulous second life at that time when conventional wisdom says she should be in a state of decline. You can do it too if you take charge of your health.

No Butts *about* It

Taking responsibility also means not smoking. You know better than anyone does all of the reasons to quit. Just remember you can do anything you put your mind to. Yes, at one time (back in the dark ages!) it was cool and sophisticated to smoke. You were encouraged to smoke and even tricked into it one way or another, with misleading health and safety claims, or relentless advertising that influenced you to put that first cigarette between your lips. But remember, you made a choice. Even after the first puff made you sick as a dog, you chose to persist. Regardless of why you began, adopt a defiant attitude and refuse to see yourself as victimized or having a "disease." Decide to be victor, not a victim. You can do it.

Since I'm a registered pharmacist, people often ask me about smoking cessation products or approaches, and here is my opinion about their effectiveness: Patches work for some people, but they are not for everybody. You really must *want* to quit in order for them to work. I've seen people use patches and continue to smoke, rationalizing that they are inhaling less tar and nicotine!

Nicotine gum is okay but some people are hooked on it, thinking chewing gum is better than inhaling. Well, maybe it is, but nicotine in any form will compromise your health.

There is prescription medication called Zyban. The same drug marketed as Wellbutrin is a treatment for depression. Does Zyban work? I personally know no success stories. It may be worth a try if your doctor agrees it's right for you. Interestingly, many insurance plans will not pay for Zyban. Yes, this seems illogical. Maybe they figure it's cheaper for them if you develop lung cancer or emphysema.

Finally, there is the cold turkey approach which many people simply can't endure. One reason it's so tough to abruptly quit is because nicotine stimulates production of serotonin, which makes you feel good. When you try to quit, your serotonin level drops and you might become moody and irritable and that's not all. You'll crave sweets and snack food, and that's why so many people end up gaining weight when they quit smoking.

Regardless of what it takes I urge you to kick the habit so you can optimize your health every way possible. You will most likely find your craving for tobacco diminishes as you improve your health and get on a regular exercise program. Taking this approach along with whatever other support you want to try will make quitting smoking a good deal easier.

Damage from smoking can be somewhat mitigated by nutritional supplementation. For example, new research[1] suggests that taking folic acid can reduce the risk of heart impairment due to smoking. At the end of a four week study, smokers who took 5 mg per day of folic acid showed dramatically improved arterial elasticity and a five point drop in blood pressure. Those given a placebo showed no change. The recommended daily dose of folic acid is just .8mg, (you need a doctor's prescription to get 1 mg tablets) but because most people eat the typical nutrient-deficient "All American" diet, it's easy to see that most people don't get nearly enough folic acid, whether or not they are smokers.

If, as a smoker, you asked your traditionally trained physician if you should take 5 mg of folic acid every day, you'd probably send him or her into a tizzy and likely be told you'd be wasting your money, or that you would be harming yourself. For the record, I take at least 5 mg of folic acid a day and I don't smoke. Does my anti-aging physician suggest I take 5 mg of folic acid a day? No. But based on my research, that's a decision I made for myself. With nutritional supplementation sometimes you have to act with educated fearlessness. I stress educated, a state most people can reach with dedication and determination.

Here are some irrefutable facts from the National Center for Health. If you smoke and are on the fence about giving up smoking this may spur you to action:

1 *Health & Healing*, January 2003, p. 5

- Each smoked cigarette burns away eight minutes of your life.
- Smoking a pack a day translates to losing a month of life each year. Smoke two packs a day and you can sacrifice 12 to 16 years if you are a lifetime smoker.
- Smoking compromises the immune system so severely that it takes at least three months to reverse the damage to your immune system once you quit.
- Smoking one pack a day depletes 500 mg. of vitamin C, more than most people absorb in one day.
- Cigarettes elevate the carbon monoxide level in the blood, which so ruthlessly competes with oxygen that it takes the circulatory system six hours to return to normal after just one cigarette.

Maybe this information strikes you to the core. I hope so. Smoking truly sucks. It sucks the life out of you.

Be Aggressive about Your Health

One hard truth we have to accept is that doctors don't know everything. Some know more than others, but no one physician knows it all. Health care professionals want to do their best but often it's not enough. In medical school and during residency, training consists primarily of the use of diagnosis, intervention, and medications to treat illnesses and to save lives. Little consideration is given to nutrition and prevention, the most basic aspects of maintaining health. Although this approach is slowly changing, it's not happening fast enough. That means you should look out for yourself. The good news is that the information is out there if you're willing to take the initiative.

Given the reality of inadequate medical school training, if you have a health problem, you owe it to yourself to learn as much as possible about your condition so you can become an informed participant in your treatment. Please understand I'm not suggesting you come off as a "know it all" after only doing a limited amount of research and study. I'm not suggesting that you tell your doctor what to do. Think "partnership." The key is informed participation. Research, information and knowledge will empower you to make intelligent choices about the treatments your doctor may suggest. Please bear in mind you don't have to obediently accept every treatment your doctor recommends. That was the way of our parents, but it's no longer appropriate. We know too much today.

Repeatedly, customers tell me they disagree with their doctor's evaluation or treatment of their condition, but they go along with it because "the doctor said so." I personally feel it's insane to hand your body over to someone, however highly credentialed, and say, "Here's my body. Do with it what you will." Never forget: It's your life, your health, and it's your body. So take responsibility for it.

Since medical training does not focus on prevention but on treating symptoms, you can expect that your doctor will attempt to "fix" your problems with medication. If you have high blood pressure a pill will bring it down. High cholesterol? A pill will lower it. There may be little or no discussion about how lifestyle choices could contribute to, or alleviate your problem. However, when you become an informed participant in your health care, it may be possible to collaborate with your doctor so the two of you can find more prudent, non-medication solutions to your ailments.

By the way, if any doctor resists your informed participation, do the obvious and find a physician who will listen to you. Your doctor is not God, but if that's the way you see him or her, face the situation and find another medical deity. There are plenty out there. Some are better listeners and more open minded than others are. Some will even pray with you if that's your inclination. You're the consumer; you have many choices.

If you are hardy and don't have a significant health problem, now's the time to make certain one doesn't develop, especially if you have a history of a particular illness in your family. Genetics may play a minor role in our lives but I don't subscribe to the theory that just because your parents had cancer or diabetes it will be your fate. Perhaps your parents didn't live a particularly healthy lifestyle, even though they thought they were doing all the right things. Perhaps they didn't drink or smoke, but they most likely ate the disastrous All-American diet, unaware of the role it played in the condition of their health.

Facing the reality that certain ailments tend to run in the family and recognizing the role of genetics and heredity, I'm nevertheless convinced that paying attention to lifestyle choices can break the chain of many seemingly inherited diseases such as diabetes, high blood pressure, heart disease, and even cancer. When it comes to health, I'm not a fatalist; you have far more control than you may think you do. You have far more control when you are aware of and abide by the following Super Keys:

- Understand that nothing is more important than super health. To have super health it's imperative to educate yourself about diet, supplements, and anti-aging strategies. The Internet, bookstores, and libraries make it easy. Your ultimate health goal should be mental and physical strength and flexibility, and vitality that will keep you vibrant and lively.
- Love and value yourself. Your mind and body are all you will ever have and they must last a long time. When you value who you are and what you have, you are less likely to abuse yourself with the wrong kind of food (and too much of it), alcohol, tobacco and neglect.
- Believe it's possible to stave off the aging process by at least 20 years. The reality is, much of the decline traditionally associated with the aging process is nothing more than the result of a lifetime of misinformation, mismanagement, lack of education, and neglect.
- Visualize early what you want your life to be like when you are 60, 70, and beyond. When you have a clear picture of your goal you will make intuitive decisions that will open doors and propel you toward your goal.
- Drink lots of water. Most people underestimate the value of adequate water consumption. Keeping your skin and cells hydrated is essential for agelessness.
- Engage in rigorous mental management and self discipline so you will do what it takes to put old on hold.

Monitor negative self talk such as "I'm too old to do that," or "I'm having a senior moment." It hastens decline. Have a varied exercise routine and do it regularly, no matter what. Your body will thank you.
- Find a physician trained in anti-aging medicine and nutrition, someone who will partner with you in the maintenance of your health. You are the consumer and if you educate yourself you can play an active role in staying healthy and extending your lifespan.
- Monitor how you are changing over time. Know what youthful attributes are important to you and constantly work to maintain them. It should be just as easy to bend and touch your toes at age 70 as it is at twenty.
- Become an astute observer of cultural attitudes toward aging and be a critical thinker about what you see and hear. Pay attention to how those closest to you may be influencing how you age. Resist pressure to conform; create your own pathway to agelessness.
- Don't retire.

The payoff is that you will get to age 60, 70 and beyond, being capable of feeling and functioning like a healthy 40 or 50-year-old. You'll be in charge of your life at a time when conventional wisdom says you should be in a state of decline, dependent on others or locked away in a nursing home, waiting to die. Agelessness is having the freedom to live the way you want to live, being able to take advantage of the choices and opportunities traditionally available only to those much younger. It's feeling like the cat that ate the canary. When I was younger I often wondered what that expression meant. Now I know, and it's wonderful. I feel like I've cheated the aging process out of an extra 20 years and it makes me smile as the cat would, if it could, after devouring the canary. I want you to experience the same feeling of satisfaction.

The Importance of Lifestyle

Dr. John W. Rowe, president of the Mount Sinai Medical Center in New York and chairman of the MacArthur Foundation Research Network on Successful Aging, maintains that how well you age is 70 percent lifestyle and 30 percent heredity. If he is correct, (and I believe he is) then clearly, lifestyle choices matter, and they matter a lot.

But I think Dr. Rowe's lifestyle/heredity ratio is conservative. I believe how well you age is closer to 80 percent lifestyle and 20 percent heredity. There are also non-identifiable environmental or social and psychological factors, too. As longevity researchers continue to uncover what contributes to healthy longevity, Dr. Rowe's lifestyle/heredity ratio might become even more favorable. The challenge is to implement the lifestyle choices that promote optimum health and the longest possible duration of youthful characteristics.

I've said that taking responsibility for your health is a choice. Some choices will work better than others will. My intent is to help you implement the ones that will work best for you. For example, what are the benefits of a restricted calorie yet highly nutritious diet? Even though the jury is still out on the value of a low-calorie, high-nutrition diet, mounting evidence shows the idea has merit.

Personally, I feel better when I don't eat a lot. I choose food carefully, paying attention to nutritional value. When I eat a high-protein power-packed breakfast and drink a lot of water during the day, I can work for hours without feeling hungry. My mind is clearer and I have an abundance of energy. If my stomach starts to gurgle, I eat some nuts that tide me over until I come home from work. Dinner is often a bowl of oatmeal laced with ground flaxseed, topped with fruit and soy milk. Don't laugh; it's yummy!

In China, people tend to live longer than in our culture. They eat a grain-based diet, using meat sparingly as a condiment to flavor the grain. They also restrain their eating. Perhaps because of economic conditions, children learn to eat until they are *almost* full and, as part of good table manners, to take less of what they want. Over the years, I've worked with many Asian pharmacists. I've always marveled at the simplicity of their food choices and how little they eat compared to Americans who can't seem to function without consuming tons of super-sized grease, sugar, and red meat.

Think about the lifestyle you are living now. Analyze it. Who is responsible for it? Who or what influences it? What needs to be changed or improved? Will you make the changes you know you should make? Do you value yourself and the health of your family enough to take charge?

Health Care Realities

The State of Health Care Today

Managed Health Care is the norm today and health care rationing is on the horizon. To successfully put old on hold, it's important to understand how the system could affect you and how you can avoid becoming a victim of either managed care or health care rationing.

The public is growing disenchanted with health maintenance organizations (HMOs) or any kind of third party insurance. Members of HMOs see consumer costs rising and the quality of health care declining. It's not your imagination that prescription prices are sharply increasing, even if you have insurance. Co-pays have reached the level of obscene, and if you think things are bad now, get ready for what is on the way. Expensive drugs will continue to appear on the market and advertised directly to consumers, creating a demand for them. Arthritis sufferers, for example, see a compelling commercial on TV showing grandpa playing ball with the grandkids, riding a bike, or dancing. They see a full color newspaper ad for a new pain relief medication and become convinced it's the answer to their prayers. This method of advertising is called "Direct to Consumer" advertising, or DTC. It is extremely expensive and adds astronomically to the cost of prescription medications. DTC is powerful; it drives ailing consumers to the doctor's office demanding a prescription for the latest magic bullet. The doctor complies with a prescription for the advertised medication, presumably first having read information supplied by the drug manufacturer's representative.

The patient, feeling victorious about having a prescription in hand for the most advanced medication, has visions of an instant cure and hurries to the pharmacy to claim the treasure. Then reality sets in. The patient's HMO doesn't want to pay for the new drug, protesting that the older, less expensive medications work as well. (And many of them do, truth be told!)

If the doctor really wants the patient to try the new medication, the physician may have to spend time convincing the HMO why the patient needs the expensive remedy. If the HMO refuses, as it often does, and the patient really wants the new drug, the patient pays full price out of pocket. It's not uncommon for a 30-day supply of a brand new wonder drug to cost several hundred dollars. Then the distraught patient wails, "Why does this prescription cost so much?" Part of the reason is the expensive and effective DTC advertising that drove the patient scurrying to the doctor's office to ask for it.

How expensive is DTC advertising? Pharmaceutical companies spent $833 million on TV ads and $460 million on print ads in 2002[2]. In breaking those figures down, companies spent $152 per lead on TV ads and $318 per lead using print media. Now you know the cost of driving a consumer to a doctor to ask for a prescription. That sounds like a lot of money just for a lead, but not to worry. Every lead that turns into a customer will help recoup the expense for the company. And it will happen. According to a *Reuters*[3] report, retiree drug costs were expected to rise 20.9 percent in 2001

2 "Internet Drug Ads Retain Their Low-Cost Edge," *iMarketing News*, February 12, 2001.

3 "Drug Benefits Costs to Jump 20% in 2001," *Reuters Health*, October 23,2000.

(and they did rise, and continue to rise) because of rising patient demand for specific advertised medications.

Now, consider the outcome when the patient pays full price for costly medication, but it fails to produce the desired relief, or causes side effects so severe that the treatment must immediately stop: It's a lot of money down the drain. Not only is your body suffering, but so is your budget. It's especially painful if you must survive on minuscule Social Security checks.

Eventually, however, HMOs do begin to pay for the newest medications but only after securing a satisfactory financial arrangement with a drug manufacturer or the government. Or, failing that, patient co-pays increase and the cost of insurance may go up. It is not uncommon to see prescription co-pays in the $50-$75 range. That may seem high, but it isn't if the full cash price for the drug is several hundred dollars.

In spite of the effectiveness of DTC advertising, this form of marketing is suspect by some segments of the public. To test DTC acceptance, www.Medscape.com conducted a 15-day poll asking, "Do you favor or oppose direct-to-consumer advertising of prescription drugs?" Of 3,416 total responses, 31 percent favored DTC and 69 percent opposed it. It is not known how many respondents were medical professionals, but it doesn't matter. DTC produces positive financial results for advertisers and that's what counts to the pharmaceutical companies, at least for now.

To be fair, when talking about the high cost of prescription drugs, other cost factors clearly come into play. For example, U.S. pharmaceutical companies give away an estimated $8 billion in free samples each year, an amount that increases eight percent a year. Drug companies provide samples to doctors who give them to low-income or indigent patients.

It's one thing to be aware of the sampling program and another to see it in practice. Recently, while in my doctor's office waiting for my appointment, at least six drug manufacturer's sales reps came in with huge shopping bags filled with medication samples. It reminded me of kids at Halloween with their trick-or-treat bags.

As the reps gave their scripted sales pitch to the nurses (not the doctor), they scooped out handfuls of free samples. Knowing what medication costs, I witnessed a good deal of money given away as if it were candy. Some of the reps appeared very young, perhaps a couple of years out of high school. There was a time when drug companies hired licensed pharmacists to visit doctors on the assumption they had the training to professionally interact with doctors and answer technical medical questions. As I listened to the young reps give their canned presentations, I couldn't help but question how much they really knew about the products they were promoting.

In addition to medical practice sampling program, some drug companies have direct "patient assistance programs" that provide one-to-three-month supplies for low-income or indigent patients. These programs gave out $500 million in drugs in 1998 and the practice continues to this day.

Another reason for the high cost of medication is the astronomical amount of money poured into research and development of many promising drugs, which often don't work as projected and are abandoned. When a new drug is effective in clinical trials, it must first pass through a lengthy and extremely expensive process of approval (or rejection) by the federal Food and Drug Administration (FDA) before marketing can proceed. This too, adds to the high cost of prescription drugs.

The best option for you is to take care of your health so you don't have to take a ride on the medication merry-go-round. Maybe you won't avoid it entirely, but more than you might think possible. Freedom from having to take medication is a priceless prize to pursue.

Health Care Rationing

Health care rationing is closing in and the older you get the more momentous this issue becomes. Rationing means if you need or want a particular medication or a surgical procedure, whether you get it may depend on a committee that weighs the pros and cons of necessity in your situation.

I recently read an article that expressed the critical need to understand the anti-aging sentiment you will experience as you get older. The title of the article is "Is it Justifiable to Ration Healthcare on the Basis of Age?"[4] The opening paragraph states: "Since healthcare is not a limitless resource, there is little doubt that rationing is required." Please note the words: "There is little doubt" that rationing is required. Until recently, talk about rationing was an issue of "may be" or "could be," not a perceived requirement. It's the process of gradualism at work and it's important to be aware of how it works and understand the impact it has on your future.

The article says it could be argued that those who have lived to a certain age (perhaps 70 years) have already lived

4 *Drug & Therapeutic Perspectives*, 16(3):14-16, 2000

most of their expected lifespan, so priority should be given to those who have not yet lived that long. It also suggests that society has a greater duty to prevent the death of the young rather than the old. Does that sound like a good idea to you? Not if you are over seventy!

The point I want to make is this: If you take responsibility for optimizing and protecting your health early on, then healthcare rationing and doing battle with cost-conscious HMOs or any insurance entity should not have to significantly concern you.

I believe that with appropriate lifestyle choices and enhancements, it's possible to considerably reduce the need for expensive medical care. You can't eliminate all health problems from your life; you can't remove the unexpected. Certainly bad things happen to good people who do all the right things. But with intelligent lifestyle choices it's possible to substantially reduce the odds of bad things happening and significantly improve your ability to have an exceptional quality of life far longer than you thought possible.

Believe in your ability to take responsibility for your health by making intelligent lifestyle choices, and there's no better time to begin than now.

Free Yourself from Fear of the Future

Scudder Investment Services surveyed 5,000 Boomers and found 82 percent feared they would face deteriorating physical health, and 66 percent worried about not having enough money.

There are two major reasons why fear of declining health runs rampant: The first is what you experience and observe through the course of your life, and the second is social conditioning. You see people all around whose health is declining, so it seems inevitable it will happen to you. And then there are the purveyors of gloom and doom who give credence to your observations.

In just one example of the latter (and there are many more), a newsletter published by an HMO states[5], "A certain amount of short-term memory loss is normal, starting as early as one's mid-forties." Where, I ask, is the scientific documentation or absolute evidence to support this claim? Imagine the Boomers who feel insecure about their health, cringing as they read such a dire prediction. It can become a self-fulfilling prophecy, giving permission to let down one's guard, inviting decline by thinking "I must be getting old" when memory lapses occur. Everyone experiences memory lapses. They are like momentary traffic jams that clear up as quickly as they come. Don't believe something will happen just because "they" say it will.

No, you are not going to accept memory loss without a fight. You are going to consistently, persistently, and intelligently work at improving your memory and do what is necessary to hold on to your mental integrity. Learn how to protect your brain and memory by reading Brain Longevity by Dharma Singh Khalsa, M.D.(listed in the Resources section) Not only will it give you hope, it will give you tools you need to take responsibility for your mental well being.

5 *Helplines*, Summer 2000, published by PacifiCare, Laguna Hills, CA

Through the years I have worked with many conscientious, bright young people. Typically, they attend school, are involved in sports, and have a significant other. Some have two jobs. They have a lot on their minds. And guess what? When there's a ball game or an exciting event coming up they sometimes forget something they are supposed to do on the job. Of course they apologize, but never once has any one attributed a memory lapse to being young. And why should they? After all, everyone forgets now and then. Young people focus on youthful concerns while old people worry about their taxes, errant kids, their marriage, health or financial security and other related issues. The stress that accompanies preoccupation at any age often results in fleeting forgetfulness. Regardless of how old (or young) someone may be, it's reasonable to expect things to slip between the cracks once in a while. So don't sweat those little memory lapses. When they happen, let them be, without fearing that you are losing it, or berating yourself for getting old. Stay strong in your belief that you can remember whatever you want. Until and unless a qualified expert diagnoses Alzheimer's or other form of dementia, believe that your memory is working well.

Fear of decline accosts you in so many ways. I've seen an ad on TV in which a Boomer-aged woman says she isn't afraid of growing old, but she is worried she won't be able to afford the cost of medication. This is both negative and destructive. The unspoken message says you will need medication as you age and that decline and deterioration are inevitable. Don't buy into it!

It would be wonderful if public service announcements assured people that if they take responsibility for achieving optimum health, they won't need to worry so much about the cost of health care. Healthy people do not rely on the health care system to stay well. Great health is not the result of visits to the doctor or taking medication. You achieve great health by what you choose to do for yourself, day by day, year in and year out. Yes, lifestyle choices matter.

Educate Yourself!

Becoming responsible for your health begins with having the proper attitude so you can educate yourself. In our culture, we want to be healthy, we talk about it and say we value health but when it comes to doing the work, we back off. In fact, we criticize those who do the work required to stay healthy by using pejoratives such as "health nut" or "health freak." This paradox needs exposure for what it is and we need to fix it.

If you are ready to do the work necessary to be and stay healthy, you may be asking, where do I start? Please do not protest you are not intelligent or educated enough to take responsibility for your health. People often protest it's too complicated. But that's nonsense. Could it be that you just don't want to be bothered or don't want to change any habits? If you are able to hold a job and function well in your everyday life, if you can remember all kinds of sports trivia and statistics, if you can surf the Internet, you are bright enough to learn anything you want. Today, self-education is easier than ever. The Internet has more than enough information to enable anyone to acquire expertise on virtually any given subject. There is no longer (if there ever was) an excuse for ignorance. If you don't know how to surf the Internet, your local library is an excellent resource. Get to know the reference librarians; they'll be happy to help you in your quest to stay healthy and vital.

Additional resources include:

- Health and lifestyle sections of bookstores abound with well-researched books by researchers, medical doctors, alternative health gurus, and ordinary individuals who have found their own cures and reinstated their health.
- Magazine racks bulge with a variety of health-related publications.
- Health food stores offer books by alternative practitioners of every kind as well as free magazines. While the free magazines are primarily advertising vehicles for products sold in health food stores, they usually contain well-researched, documented, reliable information.
- Excellent newsletters written by medical doctors are now available by subscription. Many doctors provide their own websites. (You'll find several recommended newsletters and publications in the Resources section.)

A word of caution: If you are just beginning your quest for knowledge, don't believe everything you read. Read it, but also question it. Beware of following one "guru" or known expert. Eventually you will have absorbed enough information to make good judgments about what to believe, and what to question or dismiss. As you continue to learn, your thinking and understanding will evolve and your discernment will improve. Always stay open to new information regardless of how "expert" you may become.

Partner with Your Practitioner

There are essentially two types of doctors in our health care system: Those who treat symptoms and those who work to find causes of symptoms. The former waits for patients to get sick and the latter work at keeping you well. What kind of doctor is treating you?

You can take responsibility for your health by finding a traditionally trained medical doctor who not only treats symptoms but also looks for the cause of the symptoms. The best kind of doctor you can have not only deals with your present situation but also will work with you to prevent future problems. These doctors are called alternative or integrative physicians. They have a different mindset than strictly traditional doctors about what it takes to be well. Also, they tend to encourage full involvement of patients in their health care regimen; the partnering concept covered earlier in this book.

Alternative or integrative medical doctors use the best of both traditional medicine and alternative medicine. The integrative/alternative physician is usually more open-minded than a traditional one, and is more likely to respect your thoughts about what type of treatment is appropriate for you.

If you belong to a health plan that allows a choice of doctors, call each doctor on the list and ask if he or she practices integrative or alternative medicine. You may get lucky and find one. Or, use the Internet to check out the website for ACAM, the American College for Advancement of Medicine (www.acam.org) to find an alternative physician in your area. In going over the list provided by ACAM, do not overlook physicians with a doctor of osteopathy (DO) degree. They are sometimes more prevention oriented than a physician with an MD degree.

Too Much of a Good Thing

These days, when refurbishing football stadiums they reduce the number of seats. Sports stadiums aren't getting smaller; the seats are getting larger. This is because we are getting larger. It's easy to see why so many Americans are overweight. Fast food is everywhere; restaurants of every imaginable variety and supermarkets or delis are just a few minutes away from your home or office. There is continuous and relentless exposure to advertising for ingestibles of all kinds, fueling the desire to try this or that tasty product.

On many talk and news shows, cooking segments are the norm. Note the proliferation of TV food shows and showmen, one of the more successful being Chef Emeril Lagasse. He has turned cutsey culinary uncouthness into pseudo haute cuisine. On his "food-tainment" show, his audience is worked into drooling, adoring expectation, shrieking "oohs" and "ahs" at Emeril's every "Bam!" and "Let's add a whole bulb of 'gahlic' to kick it up a notch." The feeding frenzy revs into high gear as he passes around samples of his mouth-watering creations. The food-frantic atmosphere is heightened by a "hipper than hip" live band, and one wonders when dancing girls (well upholstered, no doubt) will be added to the celebration of gluttony.

The reality is, we have been trained to eat, even when we're not hungry. We eat for emotional comfort, for social approval, for breaks while shopping, and to assuage anger, relieve boredom, or depression. We eat as much for these reasons as to satisfy real hunger.

Food abuse is more than eating too much of the wrong food at any moment of the day. It's the non-stop calorie-dense, nutritionally bankrupt "stuff" over a long period of time. That "stuff" does not promote good health but contributes to poor health. You know the culprits: grease, fried anything, refined sugar, processed, empty calories, non-nutritious drinks, and snacks. And don't forget pickled, preserved, freshly embalmed or processed meats contaminated with bacteria.

If you are hungry for something to chew on right now, digest this: According to U.S. Department of Agriculture scientists, in 2000 Americans ate 140 more pounds of food than in 1990. Do you think we are eating less in 2004? Or how about this: The average American eats 152 pounds of sugar each year. According to Coca Cola's own figures, the average teen consumes 65 gallons of its product each year. But wait, there's more: In 2002 Americans spent $115 billion on fast food. Americans now spend more than half their food budget on food outside the home. The lust for food is not abating. It's unfair and unrealistic to blame the prevailing epidemic of obesity on heredity! We have become a nation of food abusers.

The best way to take responsibility for your health is to control what you put into your mouth. Resolve to get over your affair with food. Stop watching TV food shows. Do not swap stories with friends or coworkers about how much you stuffed yourself at dinner last night. Realize that this supports, condones, and encourages over consumption. When you see a TV or print advertisement for food, look at it objectively – don't allow their enticing visuals to override your intelligence. It won't be easy; addictions are never easy to overcome. Think critically about what you are up against and decide how you are going to handle things. Constantly remind yourself how much you value your body and your life and will not deliberately abuse it.

When you try to tame the obsession of gorging, the desire for food becomes an irrational, possessive lover. When you take on an "I don't love you anymore" mindset about eating when you are not really hungry, food becomes a stalker, constantly tempting you to eat, whispering "try this, just one little bite won't matter." Recognize the temptation for what it is and deal with it firmly.

Speaking of culprits, I was recently walking by a food court in a shopping mall and took note of what people were consuming. One plate in particular caught my eye. On it was a mound of deep brown, deep-fried whatever. It looked like a pile of turtle turds. The person devouring it was obese. When was the last time you had a plate of greasy, indescribable yummies? Don't do it again! I'll report you to the grease police and commit you to a vegetarian health spa for recovering food or grease-a-holics. (Just kidding. I would never do that to you. We all have dietary lapses now and then.) I think fast food grease is addictive. One of my relatives says he has to go to a fast food place at least once a week for his grease fix. He's kidding, I hope, but ingesting high amounts of grease, possibly on its way to being rancid, is a way of life for too many of us.

Now that I've reamed the All-American preoccupation with gorging, I feel better and I'm ready to get back on a positive track. Another Super Key to good health and longevity may be the opposite of gluttony: fasting. A concept as old as the Bible, fasting is now gaining acceptance among mainstream medical practitioners. Dr. Stephen Sinatra, in his newsletter, The *Sinatra Health Report*, March 2001, says that fasting, in addition to other health benefits, doubles growth hormone (HGH) levels. Human growth hormone is a substance you have when you are young and is responsible for youthful characteristics. Over time, HGH production slowly declines, resulting in signs of advancing age. It's possible to restore youthful qualities with injections of supplemental human growth hormone, but it is not without risks. HGH can accelerate cell division, possibly putting anyone who takes it at an increased risk of cancer. If fasting a day or two a week can naturally boost your own production of HGH, it seems miraculous and well worth a try. You can learn more about HGH in *Grow Young with HGH* by Dr. Ronald Klatz. He gives resources for HGH, anti-aging therapies, and a list of physicians who specialize in anti-aging medicine. (You'll find Resources at the end of this book.

Let me digress for a moment with a word of caution about over-the-counter products that purport to be HGH or contain HGH "releasers." Real HGH is an injectible product available only on prescription and its use must be carefully monitored by a physician. Non-prescription HGH releasers are supposed to help the body make its own HGH. If you were to ask me what I think about non-prescription HGH products I'd say they are obscenely expensive and not worth your money. If you are determined to try a releaser product, do so in a rational manner. Before using the product, be it sprays, tablets or powder, have a physician order a blood test to determine your level of Igf-1, which is an indicator of your current level of HGH. After taking the releaser product for six months, have another test for Igf-1. Your physician will quickly be able to tell you if the product has made a difference.

Back to fasting. Fasting doesn't mean having to starve. One or two days a week you can fast on juices as well as water to keep you up and running. Fast on a day you don't go to work or do anything too strenuous. If you have a juicer, you can have an enjoyable, beneficial fast using a variety of fresh fruits and vegetables. But fasting is not for everyone. If you are diabetic or have other health problems, check with your physician first.

I believe another Super Key is an obvious yet underestimated one: water consumption. An amazing number of people don't like water. Yet, your body is composed of 80 to 90 percent water. Every cell depends on having enough water to function optimally. If you don't constantly replenish the water your body uses to process food, eliminate toxins, and keep it operating as intended, you will have difficulty maintaining even minimal good health. The value of adequate water consumption is undeniable. Those who drink volumes of water remain like beautiful juicy plums and those who don't shrivel up. I'll discuss more about water later.

Stamp Out Food Abuse

Everyone makes poor food choices occasionally. The occasional faux pas won't destroy your health. Once in a while is not the same as day in and day out, year after year, of constant, systematic, unrelenting food abuse. Are you a "systematic overeater?" If so, admit that you have some serious issues with food. That's the first step to taking control. But you may protest, you don't inflict food abuse on the one and only body you will ever have; you just do what everybody else does. You just eat the traditional, daily, All-American diet and what's wrong with that? Well, a lot!

Look, you can't treat your body - your temple — with disdain and disrespect for 50 years, stuffing into it the worst elements of the All-American diet and expect your body to run like a trouble-free Mercedes for the next fifty. Consider that 90 percent of the money spent on food in America goes to buying processed food[6]. What is processed food? It's anything created in a corporate food laboratory. You buy it in boxes, cartons, jars, packets, cans and bags. It's frozen, instant, heat 'n eat. In my opinion, calling it food is being charitable. Most of it is nutritionally worthless. Dog food, as bad as much of it is, even for dogs, may be more nutritious.

---

6 *Fast Food Nation* by Eric Schlosser, p.121

You can change your diet if you really want to. You weren't born loving pizza, greasy burgers, and high calorie "pseudo" foods such as French fries, buffalo wings, fried mozzarella sticks, deep fried Twinkies and even deep fried Snickers bars. Once you make a commitment to your health and make the lifestyle changes that will enable you to put old on hold, you will eagerly want to eat what's good for you. You will treat your body with respect. You will learn the magic and joy of eating to live instead of living to eat which will eliminate the practice of ignoring "full" signals. Often, it isn't all in what we eat but how much and when.

Along the way on your resolve to change your way of eating you will suffer relapses, and that's okay as long as you stay focused and don't use the lapses as an excuse to give up. It's okay to have an occasional dessert, piece of chocolate or glass of wine. It's okay to have breakfast at McDonald's once in a while. The key word is occasional. By the way, here's a tip about drinking alcohol: When you have that occasional glass of wine or beer, follow up with at least one or two glasses of water and a high potency B-complex tablet or capsule. Alcohol is dehydrating and robs the body of vitamins. This way you help to quickly pay for your momentary indiscretion. Caution: Don't think you can drink a six-pack of beer and follow up with a gallon of water and a several B vitamins. That's abuse with a stupid attitude!

The Classic Signs of Food Abuse

After eating a greasy hamburger or any concoction dripping with grease, preservatives and chemicals, it's not uncommon for your stomach to complain loudly, and a little later experience gas, bloating, pain, and constipation. When that happens, listen to the wisdom of your body and stop the abuse. Don't continue to eat what your taste buds love but your stomach hates.

Food abuse is encouraged in TV commercials. Don't believe the ads that suggest you can eat mountains of indigestible material masquerading as food and then pacify the resultant symptoms by popping a pill or drinking an antacid mixture. That is wrong headed. Your body can tolerate food abuse for just so long before you develop serious problems. You will eventually experience intestinal distress. Your liver will begin acting up. Your cholesterol will stock pile. Your arteries will start to clog. Your gall bladder will rebel. You may even develop gastroesophogeal reflux disease (GERD), and it is very painful. If not that, you make yourself vulnerable to a host of other disorders.

If you want to put old on hold, ignore TV commercials that encourage you to trick your body with pills or potions. They simply don't work.

Why We Abuse Food

The ingestible (and often indigestible) high fat, low nutrition fare of the All-American diet becomes the basis of what most people consume. I call these food items "ingestible" because they are manufactured food products resulting from scientific tinkering in corporate laboratories. Good, natural ingredients are processed and re-engineered to not only taste terrific but to also provide emotional satisfaction. There's an insidious element to these manufactured foods; the emotional satisfaction is there, but not the physical satisfaction. Too often, eating one créme-filled donut or salty greasy chip isn't enough. You crave more, and when that happens it means the food scientists have achieved their goal: They have created something that sells, and sells, and sells some more! To make it even more tempting, beloved and respected celebrities, cartoon characters, or actors posing as experts advertise the products on TV. Obediently, viewers rush out to buy these "food" products. Obesity, anyone? Is there any doubt why so many people in our culture become food abusers? And by the way, do some over-eaters have a hidden agenda, an unconscious desire for punishment?

Enticing, full-color newspaper ads, introductory offers and supermarket specials support TV advertising. Larger-than-life images of palate-pleasing products have your mouth watering in anticipation. You clip the coupons and try new products. Once you put a morsel in your mouth, your taste buds scream for more. However much you eat, it's never enough, so you chow down the whole box or bag. Isn't science wonderful? Sure it is, but when it comes to food, what Mother Nature produces is far superior.

The Supermarket: Temple of Temptations

Seductive food ads would be meaningless without a place to buy the products. Take a look at the layout of your favorite market and scrutinize the mile-long aisle of shelves loaded with breakfast cereals. Just about every home in America starts the day with puffed, popped, flaked, or shredded cereals fortified with vitamins because processing destroys the nutrients originally provided by Mother Nature. What makes them appealing are taste, texture, and unquestioned tradition. The major reason people continue to buy these products is habit. When my daughter was little, after watching a TV commercial for corn flakes, she asked me to buy a box. I said no but she was relentless and I finally gave in. Guess what? In her innocent, innate wisdom, she "yukked" at the soggy sloppy mess in her bowl and never again asked for corn flakes or any other pseudo cereal product.

People leave for a day of work after eating a bowl of commercial cereal then feel hungry for real food a few hours later. Their blood sugar, having spiked after the surge of sugar in the cereal, has plummeted. They are now craving donuts and coffee for an energy pickup. At the same time, kids are sent off to school, loaded with enough carbohydrate from breakfast cereal or toaster pastries to send a rocket into space. When they can't sit still or concentrate, behavioral specialists decide the sugar-shocked kids have Attention Deficit Disorder (ADD). The cure is a narcotic drug that turns kids into obedient, submissive zombies, at least until they become teenagers. Certainly, nutritional deficiency is not the only reason youngsters exhibit ADD or ADD-like behavior, but it's a significant reason.

Judging by the number of prescriptions I fill for Ritalin, Dexedrine, and Adderall, one would think there was an epidemic of maladjusted or brain-damaged children in our country. Wouldn't it make more sense to examine, and improve the diet before relying on a prescription drug? If that doesn't work, at least it would get kids started on a course of sensible food choices. It's never too soon to begin sound nutrition. After all, you begin to age the moment you are born.

When I was a child, ADD was unknown. I don't recall classrooms in chaos with kids unable to behave or concentrate. Children sat in their seats and learned what the teacher taught. The few students who decided to demonstrate "attention deficit" behavior cooled their heels in the principal's office until the misbehavior disappeared. At that time, sugary, lifeless breakfast cereals were not a staple in every home. During the depression years, breakfast was a cheese spread (protein) on whole wheat bread (not processed white fluff). Or maybe even eggs, if the budget allowed. From a nutrition standpoint, it was a lot better than what most children from poor and affluent homes alike, now eat every morning.

Although the nutritional content of breakfast cereals has improved in recent years, don't kid yourself — much of it is still pseudo food. It has little more nutritional value than shredded or flaked cardboard or puffed Styrofoam, regardless of what advertising says about vitamin fortification. Since I know it will be very difficult for many families to give up breakfast cereals, I thought perhaps I could suggest the names of a couple of less offensive products. But on further reflection, I thought, I don't waste my money on this stuff and I'm not going to suggest that others do so. If you want to use bran type cereals, at least read the labels carefully and decide for yourself if the high carbohydrate, low protein, or high fat and minimal vitamin content of the products is worth the price. When you read labels, you will surely conclude that for your breakfast you can do better with nutritious, whole grain bread (which still has its vitamin and mineral content) slathered with cottage cheese or almond nut, or soy butter and a drizzle of honey.

You might consider eating oatmeal, which cooks faster than you can pop a pastry into the toaster, and you'll then have something nutritious at a fraction of the cost. And for a fast dose of protein, how about eggs? I know they aren't recommended if you have high cholesterol, and experts warn us not to eat more than a couple a week. But it all depends on which experts you listen to. I am convinced eggs are not deserving of the bad press they have received. They are an excellent source of protein, and if you are counting carbs, you couldn't ask for much better. I love eggs and eat them every day, and my cholesterol is low. Eggs don't have to be boring and there are dozens of ways to prepare them.

Miles of Not So Incredible Edibles

Let's go back to the supermarket: With your new awareness, look at the mile-long aisle beckoning you with all the snack foods: cakes, donuts, the chips, the sodas, the deceptive low fat but high carbohydrate nutritionally worthless goodies. Now you are ready to shop more carefully. Read the labels. If you can't pronounce all of the ingredients listed on a container, you probably don't want it in your body. Spend your money on real food that will help you put old on hold. People often think they can't afford to eat quality food. They could if they started reading labels and stopped spending money on ingestible junk.

Some people (not you, of course) actually forego breakfast cereal and instead, have donuts and caffeinated soda or coffee for breakfast (or other junk too horrible to mention). Just spend a few moments at your local convenience store in the morning and watch what people buy on their way to work. Constant overload of sugar and caffeine really abuses your body. Those chronic coffee and caffeinated soda junkies (this includes diet soda as well) and donut dunkers can forget about putting old on hold. They will go through blood sugar surges and slumps all day and this takes a toll. They don't realize it but they are or are begging to be the diabetics of tomorrow.

Take into consideration that it's our free enterprise system at work enticing you into making diet choices. It's called buy, buy, buy. Love yourself enough to resist! The purpose of creating an ingestible or processed food product (or any product, for that matter) is to produce a profit. That's the primary concern of our corporations. It's not concern for nutritional value, or your health. It's profit, pure and simple. That's okay; profit makes our economy work. But think before you purchase. Our system produces extraordinary abundance that is to be envied; yet we are not nearly as healthy or health conscious as we could or should be. The variety of choices available allows you to make intelligent choices about food. Simply be aware and *think* when deciding what you will put into your mouth.

The pharmacy where I work is located in a supermarket. I see shopping carts piled with red meat, processed, fatty foods, chips, sodas, frozen pizzas and similar tongue-tickling delights. I see loaves of bread that rival Kleenex for whiteness, softness, and nutritional value. I see boxes of breakfast cereals devoid of significant food value, nutritionally worthless donuts, snack foods and perhaps a head of iceberg lettuce and a couple of tasteless hothouse tomatoes with little or no nutritional value. It doesn't take a rocket scientist to understand the need for medications to control high blood pressure, high cholesterol and gastrointestinal upset problems.

It is unfortunate that those with the most pronounced medical problems don't make the connection between their condition and what they consume. They believe they are eating a healthy well-balanced diet because they eat a variety of attractive, tasty ingestibles. They rationalize that just about everyone else eats the same thing, so it must be okay. But it's not okay, and yes, just about everybody does eat the same corporate-created diet. The result is an epidemic of obesity, high blood pressure, high cholesterol, diabetes, gastrointestinal troubles, and other conditions that appear to have no definitive cause.

Buy Now, Pay Later

Here's the reality: If you depend on a nutritionally unsound diet day in and day out over many years, your ability to put old on hold will be difficult and probably impossible. You will have damage to undo before you can move forward. It's time to get a new attitude. Change your diet starting today.

Regardless of your age or state of health, I bet I can predict what you are thinking: "*Give up what I love to eat for a benefit I may not realize until far into the future? You have to be kidding! Give up my two-martini business lunches, breakfast meats, no more greasy casseroles, hot dogs, chips or cheese dips? Give it all up for salads and soy burgers? No way. I feel great. There's nothing wrong with my health. I'm going to be just fine.*" Sorry, you won't be fine. You'll be sick and old just when you could be starting a healthy, vigorous second life. You can't get away with bad food habits if you want to put old on hold. Decide to change your life right now. Start small; make your changes little by little and keep on going.

Supplements and Why We Need Them

It's not easy to turn away from what you've been happily eating for years without question. To do so means you are fighting not only deeply ingrained habits and preferences of your taste buds but family customs and social tradition. However, you must take charge of your health. A food consumption study conducted in the mid-1980s by the U.S. Department of Agriculture evaluated the food intake of 21,500 people over three days. Not one person met the recommended daily allowance (RDA) for the top ten nutrients, and the RDA set by the government is unrealistically low. In case you are wondering, diets have not improved since then.

Perhaps you've already tempted debilitating old age with poor food choices. Most people have. But you are not doomed particularly if you mend your ways early enough (that means now). The body is incredibly forgiving and often responds miraculously to tender, aggressive, loving care. If in reading this book you were to discover that you've fallen prey to food abuse, you can help compensate by taking supplements.

But brace yourself: If or when you ask a traditionally trained physician if you should take a vitamin supplement, chances are the doctor will say, "If you eat a well-balanced diet, you don't need vitamin supplements. You are throwing your money away." I would like to ask doctors to explain their definition of a well-balanced diet. They probably live on the same deficient All-American diet as most of their patients. Many know relatively little about optimum nutrition, because, as already mentioned, medical school gives short shrift to nutrition and wellness education. This is slowly changing but we have a long way to go. Since the American Medical Association recently changed its long-standing opposition to vitamin supplements and now recommends at least one multi-vitamin a day, some doctors may change their attitude. But I wouldn't count on it happening en masse any time soon. Set-in-concrete thinking takes time to change.

Harvard University has a new division of Complementary and Alternative Medicine, and many other universities are implementing alternative medicine programs, including a Program in Integrative Medicine at the University of Arizona Health Sciences Center. Even hospitals are getting involved with alternative treatments. Beth Israel Medical Center in New York has a center that offers homeopathic and chiropractic therapy. Herbal medications for depression are offered at the University of Pittsburgh Medical Center. This is not leaps and bounds progress, but it is real progress, so let's be grateful and hope for more in the future.

Supplementation Is a Personal Choice

Even though many physicians resist change, and still believe that if you eat a well balanced diet you don't need supplements, this new awakening in health care helps explain why the more traditionally trained doctors recommend supplements, albeit cautiously. It's now officially okay to do so; the possibility of being stigmatized as an irrational health nut has now been somewhat mitigated. If there is one thing medical practitioners fear, it's the scorn of their peers. They consult with each other about what's okay and what's not. A mainstream doctor doesn't want to come off as a kook by colleagues. A good example is what happened to Nobel Prize winner Linus Pauling. He was a respected and celebrated anti-war activist until he made known his controversial views on the benefits of high dose vitamin C. After that, his status as a credible scientist diminished in the medical community. Although his research on vitamin C is now accepted, he never regained his once revered position among many of his peers.

What Your Doctor or Pharmacist May Not Tell You

Supplements are critical for those taking prescription medications. For example, oral contraceptives, taken by many Boomers, deplete the body of vitamin B-6, folic acid, vitamin B-12, vitamin C, and the minerals zinc and magnesium. What is the significance of these depletions? For one thing, depletion of vitamin B-6 reduces synthesis of serotonin, which can result in depression and anxiety. Could that explain why so many women on oral contraceptives also take antidepressants? Depletion of vitamin B-6 also reduces synthesis of melatonin, which can cause sleep difficulties, and raises homocysteine levels, which can damage arteries, increase plaque formation, and boost the risk of cardiovascular disease.

Diuretics or water pills can deplete potassium. So-called "loop diuretics" such as furosemide can deplete calcium and magnesium. Calcium loss is significant for older women at risk of osteoporosis, especially in their later years.

A substance called coenzyme Q10 (usually referred to as CoQ10) protects the heart and is vital to cellular energy production. It is so important that a major manufacturer of cholesterol-lowering statin drugs is considering adding CoQ10 to these drugs because statins tend to deplete it. Yet, how many people taking these anti-cholesterol drugs know enough or are encouraged to supplement their diet with CoQ10. It is available without a prescription. Many people take cardiovascular drugs, which include metoprolol, atenolol, pindolol, propranolol (to mention just a few) all of which cause CoQ10 depletion. Potential depletion problems manifest as congestive heart failure, high blood pressure, and generalized low energy. Unfortunately, we don't always get the whole picture. This is another example of why we need to take responsibility for our health.

Then, too, many diseases can contribute to, or worsen nutrient deficiencies. For example, diabetics don't assimilate zinc very well, yet it's necessary for healing wounds. Diabetics may also be deficient in magnesium and chromium. If you take anticonvulsants, you too may experience nutrient depletion. For example, the drug Dilantin can deplete biotin, calcium, folic acid, vitamin B1, vitamin B12, vitamin D and vitamin K. Other anticonvulsant medications can cause similar losses. Anyone who takes medication on a regular basis should have a copy of *Drug-Induced Nutrient Depletion Handbook* by Ross Pelton, et al. This should be a resource in every home, particularly if serious health problems exist, requiring continuous use of different medications.

What I've mentioned here is just the tip of the iceberg. It's not my intention to give you a crash course on nutrition, but I want you to be aware of how some prescription medications can adversely affect your health. If you want to put old on hold, take responsibility: Understand what medications not only can do *for* you, but *to* you. Do your research.

The Anti-Aging Supplements: Your Secret Weapon

You may be wondering what supplements are needed to put old on hold? Just about everything! But how do you know which ones to take? Books, magazines, newsletters, and the Internet abound with information about good nutrition and supplements. If you need a push in the right direction, you'll find some of my favorites in the Resources section. But I won't reinvent the wheel by summarizing in-depth information available from experts more qualified than I am. My job is to present you with enough information about diet and supplements to motivate you to start educating yourself in earnest.

Before I get more specific here is some general information about buying supplements. When vitamin supplements first started appearing on the market, a worthwhile supplement came from an "organic" source. Everything had to be natural. My main source of nutrition information at that time was *Prevention* magazine when its founder, J. I. Rodale, was at the helm. As an organic farmer, his recommendations favored organic products. For many years, I tried to stay with organic or natural products, but as my education broadened, I concluded that other factors matter as well. I believe it's important to buy supplements from companies that have been in business a long time, have rigid quality controls and are actively engaged in research.

As you further your education, you will learn to make good choices. The worst decision you can make is not to do anything at all for fear of making a wrong one. If you are not taking supplements now and want to start, you can't go wrong if you purchase them from your pharmacy or a health food store with a good reputation.

The following are supplements that I believe are critical for putting old on hold.

- First on the list are antioxidants. Earlier in this book I mentioned the Free Radical Theory of aging and why it makes sense to me. Very simply, this theory holds that oxidants called free radicals cause aging, which result from the metabolism of food and from toxins. Free radicals are highly reactive and they can attack healthy cells and DNA, weakening collagen and contributing to various diseases. As you age, your body becomes more vulnerable to the effects of free radicals. I firmly believe a major cause of the "oldness" associated with aging is a result of free radical damage.

- Fortunately, you can supplement your diet with antioxidants that include vitamins C, E, CoQ10, and alpha lipoic acid. These are *my* favorites, but remember, these are not recommendations. I know what works for me and encourage you to educate yourself about what's right for you.
- Alpha lipoic acid. This may be more potent than either ginkgo or vitamin E in protecting the brain. Because it's the only antioxidant that can easily reach into the brain, it's considered useful in preventing damage from a stroke. It's been used for some time in Europe for supplementary treatment of diabetes and neurological diseases. One of alpha lipoic acid's amazing attributes is its ability to regenerate vitamins C and E after the C and E have been scavenging free radicals. This provides these antioxidants with enough oomph to continue fighting still more free radicals.
- Ginkgo biloba. I take it every day and believe it plays a major role in maintaining the integrity of my memory and cognitive ability. Ginkgo networks with vitamins C, E, and alpha lipoic acid, providing a super-effective free radical fighting machine.
- CoQ10. This supplement is enormously protective of the brain as well as the heart. CoQ10 recycles vitamin E and works with vitamin E in the skin, protecting against UV radiation. Research on this supplement show it is vitally important to maintain health and longevity.
- Networking antioxidants appear to be involved in preventing and combating gum disease. (Nearly half of

Americans aged 65 to 74 have severe periodontal disease. Bacteria in the mouth associated with gum disease may be linked to heart disease, artery blockage, and stroke.)

Additional Information on Supplements

- People who take vitamin E are 40-50 percent less likely to die of cancer or heart disease than those who don't. Men who take vitamin E are 42 percent less likely to die of prostate cancer.
- Antioxidants can keep cells youthful by preventing the accumulation of a waste product called lipofuscin. "Age spots" on the hands are one manifestation of lipofuscin.
- Antioxidants may be able to block activation of viral genes, keeping various viruses dormant.
- Polyphenols found in wine protect not only against heart disease but also against certain cancers, Alzheimer's, and macular degeneration. Moderate wine drinkers tend to live longer than teetotalers do. (Remember to follow up with a glass of water for each glass of wine consumed and a B-complex vitamin for each session of indulgence!)
- Vitamin C's ability to stimulate collagen production and thus strengthen connective tissue is a vital part of the body's defense against viruses.
- Men can cut their risk of heart attack by 45 percent simply by taking 300 mg of vitamin C a day, according to a UCLA study.

- Antioxidants have a profound role in preventing cancer because they can switch on and off the genes that control cell growth.

The above information is gleaned from a new book, *The Antioxidant Miracle* by Lester Packer, Ph.D., director of the Packer Lab at the University of California, Berkeley. It is "must reading" if you are serious about understanding the Free Radical Theory of aging. See the Resources section.

Here is more useful information about vitamin C:

- Most people who have diabetes have a greater need for vitamin C than the average person.
- Smoking depletes vitamin C.
- Long-term supplementation with vitamin C is found to reduce the risk of developing cataracts.
- Vitamin C causes wounds to heal 40-50 percent faster than without it.
- Low vitamin C intake is a risk factor for asthma.
- Vitamin C is a natural antihistamine.
- High doses of vitamin C suppress the symptoms of HIV/AIDS and can significantly reduce the tendency for secondary infections.

Other Possible Supplements

- Soy and whey. I like them for their protein value because I don't eat a lot of meat, red or white.
- Calcium, magnesium, folic acid, bioflavonoids, the entire B complex family.

- SAM-e, short for S-adenosylmethionine. It's a naturally occurring compound with multiple benefits. It's used to treat Parkinson's disease, multiple sclerosis, and migraine headaches. It has been shown to stimulate cartilage growth and may reverse the underlying causes of osteoarthritis. Clinical trials have demonstrated SAM-e has analgesic and anti-inflammatory effects. It is comparable to non-steroidal anti-inflammatories such as ibuprofen and naproxen without the side effects. I take it as a preventive measure.
- Indole-3-carbinol. Based on the studies I've seen, it shows promise of protecting against breast cancer. My doctor, who practices integrative medicine, is especially keen about using this supplement.
- Bran and psyllium. Fiber plays a vital role in the ability to put old on hold. I can't stress enough the importance of a daily bowel movement. Toxic buildup from stored waste material is not healthy. A clean intestine will go a long way toward preventing or alleviating many health problems. If you don't want to take bran and psyllium every day try eating breads baked by the Alvarado Street Bakery (www.alvaradostreetbakery.com). A couple of slices a day of their California Complete Protein bread or Barley bread works wonders. If not in stores in your area, order online. It's been said death begins with chronically clogged intestines. Believe it, and make sure it's not your problem!
- A "greens" supplement such as Vitamineral Green that is a freeze-dried mixture of green veggies, grasses and

minerals. I don't think people get enough greens even in the best diets.

- Glucosamine and chondroitin in conjunction with MSM (methylsulfonylmethane) for relief of joint pain, for lubrication and restoration of cartilage. When these supplements work, they often do so with dramatic results. It's important to be patient when expecting relief from Glucosamine. Those who use it say it can take up to a year to work but it is well worth the wait. And it doesn't have the nasty side effects of ibuprofen and other prescription anti-inflammatory drugs. I take glucoasmine and MSM as a preventive measure.

Water, Water Everywhere, But Who Stops to Drink?

Do you like water? If not, why not? Do you drink an adequate amount of water every day? What is adequate? A friend of mine carries around a pint bottle of water and sips it occasionally. She is convinced she drinks enough water. No, it's not nearly enough!

I personally believe many problems traditionally associated with old age are not the result of the aging process, but the result of dehydration. When I counsel customers about their medication, I routinely ask how much water they consume. More times than not they say they don't like water, that it makes them nauseous, bloated or that it makes them urinate too often. (Thank goodness for indoor plumbing!)

I recall vividly an older woman complaining that her saliva was too thick and she had sores in her mouth. I asked how much water she drank and, predictably, she said, "I don't drink water. It makes me sick to my stomach." No amount of scolding would have encouraged her to drink more water. Sadly, she was drying up from the inside out. This woman was mummifying herself. Unfortunately, she didn't realize that by not drinking water she was shortening her life. She is not an exception. Few people recognize the centrality of water in their diet. Something to think about: If you are not a water drinker, have health problems, and you start to drink large amounts of water, it's reasonable to expect you may feel nauseous because you are stirring up the stored toxins. If you continue to drink water, expect to feel sick until your body is back in balance.

How Much Water is Enough?

If you are sedentary and spend a good deal of your day in air-conditioned rooms, you will need less water than if you are outside working hard and sweating. But you still need water! I try to consume at least a gallon a day. Another rule of thumb is to calculate half an ounce of water per pound of body weight. Just so you know, I don't drink tap water. I drink steam distilled water when possible. I simply don't trust tap water for purity and I want my water free of chemicals.

While some water contaminants result from natural sources (pathogens from wildlife and toxic minerals that leach from ground minerals), my concern is sewage, industrial waste, pesticide runoff, illegal dumping, and just plain defective inconsistent treatment. I don't think purification systems in any municipality are completely trustworthy.

In 1993, Milwaukee, Wisconsin, experienced a disastrous outbreak of a gastrointestinal disease resulting from a pathogen called cryptosporidium in the water supply. A large number of people became sick, many hospitalized, and some died. In 1995, a study conducted by the Natural Resources Defense Council declared some 25,000 public water systems failed to meet EPA standards. That means that millions of Americans were and perhaps are still drinking water improperly treated to remove lead, parasites, and bacteria, to mention just a few potentially harmful contaminants. These and other revealing reports have been a real wake-up call for me, bolstering my resolve to avoid tap water whenever possible.

Adding chlorine and fluoride to tap water concerns me. I can accept chlorine in the water because it's necessary for purification. However, that's not an endorsement of chlorine. Chlorine reacts with naturally occurring organic matter, resulting in the formation of trihalomethanes (THMs), known to cause rectal and bladder cancers and birth defects. I know all the arguments in favor of fluoridated water, but I don't buy them. Adding a toxic substance to a community's water supply, regardless of noble intent, doesn't make sense to me.

Exposure to fluoride occurs in toothpaste, mouthwash, chewing gum, children's vitamins often given from birth, and other sources of which you are probably unaware. How much is too much? How can you know how much you are swallowing when it comes from so many different sources? I don't know of any study that proves fluoride does not accumulate in the body and where it could do irreparable harm. Do not misunderstand or underestimate the power of fluoride; it is not a benign substance. A major use for sodium fluoride is to kill roaches. While valuable, minuscule amounts may be good for preventing cavities in the teeth of children or preventing osteoporosis in older people, I don't think it's wise to mass-medicate entire communities. I often wonder if exposure to excessive fluoride plays a role in the development of Alzheimer's or other common degenerative diseases. Perhaps one day we will find out.

You may be wondering what kind of water you should drink. As I've already mentioned, I prefer steam-distilled water. Spring water is a second choice. Anything labeled "purified" or "drinking water" is not okay. Purified water is just tap water cleaned up. I am aware some expensive brands of bottled water are simply purified tap water and found to contain unacceptable levels of bacteria. You take a chance no matter what brand you buy. I still think bottled water is better than tap water, particularly if your city is delivering sanitized waste water, as had been suggested and rejected (I hope forever) in my area. Then there is well water for those who live in the suburbs. Get it tested often. Pollution is closing in!

What about gadgets you attach to your faucet? Or pitcher-type filter systems? They improve the taste but probably don't get rid of fluoride, pesticides, bacteria and poisons such as lead, mercury, or arsenic. Lead-based paints are no longer used but drinking water may still be fed through lead pipes. It is estimated that over half of the cities in the United States have lead or lead-lined pipes in municipal systems. If you are considering a home purification system, do your homework. Ask for documentation as to its efficiency.

If you are determined to use tap water, at least have it tested by a private laboratory. In addition to knowing what's in the water sample submitted you will gain an indication of whether your house plumbing is adding anything dangerous or harmful to your water supply. The safest water to drink is water that has been steam distilled. It's available in supermarkets along with all the fancy, flavored, expensive branded waters of questionable quality.

The Wonders of Water Consumption

I truly believe water "rules" as nature's wonder drug. Here are some benefits you will derive from adequate water consumption:

- Water is a natural appetite suppressant. Cold water seems to work best for this purpose. Try it when you feel hungry, particularly if you ate just a short time before. Hunger pangs are often a manifestation of hidden thirst. A woman asked me about the effectiveness of weight loss products because nothing she tried had worked. When she said she was always hungry, I asked how much water she drank. "Hardly any. It's overrated," she snapped. When I told her hunger was often a sign of hidden thirst, she grinned, narrowed her eyes, and smirked, "Yeah, right." Some people want to hear only what they want to hear, even if it's wrong information. Maybe she believes the earth is flat, too.

- Water helps the body burn stored fat. When water intake is inadequate, fat deposits increase. This is because, without enough water, the kidneys don't work up to their capacity. When this occurs, the liver has to take over some of the load. One of the liver's duties is to burn stored fat. If it is overloaded by having to take on work the kidneys should be doing, the liver burns less fat and consequently more fat remains stored in the body. Inadequate water consumption is probably a contributing factor in our nation's obesity rate.
- Adequate water consumption is a great treatment for water retention. When the body doesn't get enough water, it feels endangered and holds on to as much water as it can. This shows up as swollen ankles, legs, and hands. Prescription diuretics offer a temporary solution, forcing out stored water but it will also eliminate essential nutrients as well. As a result, the body senses a threat to survival and will replace the lost water as quickly as possible. The water retention then starts all over again. The best way to avoid water retention is to give your body plenty of water. Only then is stored water released. Regularly drinking water also helps to get rid of excess salt. The more salt you consume, the more water your body needs to dilute it. Fortunately, it's easy to get rid of excess salt, just drink more water.
- Disregard claims that it's not necessary to drink at least eight glasses of water daily as long as you drink other liquids. Water is water and you cannot replace it with

coffee, soda or other beverages. Bear in mind that if you don't drink water regularly you lose your natural thirst *and* taste for it. If that has happened to you, learn to like water again by flavoring each glassful with something like cranberry or lemon juice, gradually eliminating the flavoring.

- Since water is the key to fat metabolism, if you are overweight, you need more water than a thin person.
- Water helps maintain muscle tone by giving muscles their natural ability to contract and by preventing dehydration. Adequate water also helps prevent sagging skin after weight loss.

Be kind to your body; give it the water it wants and needs to function optimally. It will reward you by helping you to stay a juicy plum instead of becoming a dried-up prune. If you have a medical problem, consult your physician before changing your water intake.

Can Water Hold a Cure?

In *Your Body's Many Cries for Water,* F. Batmanghelidj, M.D., explains the role of water in alleviating medical problems most commonly treated with medications. He maintains that water is useful treatment for just about everything from arthritis to depression. Whether his claims are true or not, I don't know. But he does present some intriguing ideas and testimonials from those "cured" with water.

For example, he maintains that heartburn pain indicates a state of dehydration and relates how he successfully used water to treat a patient with this problem. A young man was suffering with agonizing stomach pain and had taken several cimetidine tablets and a whole bottle of antacid without relief. (Let me digress for a moment to state that it's not uncommon for those in search of relief for stomach distress to consume an entire bottle of antacid on a regular basis. That is an example of real health abuse!)

After determining that the patient didn't have a perforated ulcer, the doctor had him drink a total of three glasses of water, which resulted in complete remission of pain in a short period of time. I personally have heard testimonies about the effectiveness of water in treating stomach pain, but unless you experience it yourself, this cure, or you could say simple treatment, could be difficult to believe. After all, water is just water, isn't it?

At work one evening, a young woman handed me a prescription for ranitidine, commonly used to treat heartburn. I asked her how much water she drinks and she replied, "As little as possible. Water makes me sick." I told her about Dr. Batmanghelidj's book but she wasn't interested. She didn't like water and wasn't going to drink any. Anyway, how could something as simple as water stop stomach pain? A closed mind is a terrible thing. This unfortunate young woman is on a path to serious health problems as a result of her stubborn, earth is flat attitude.

What Every Consumer Needs to Know about Medications

At the beginning of this book, I may have mentioned that I hold unconventional and controversial views and that should be evident by now! Here's one of them: You can't put old on hold if you take a lot of unnecessary medication, whether prescription or over-the-counter (OTC) variety. That's a strong statement, but bear with me as I explain. Remember, I am speaking from my experience. You may not agree with the way I see things. I respect your right to disagree, yet I ask you to have an open mind about my point of view.

From my perspective, there are two types of medication: (1) Those needed for conditions such as seizures or infections or some medical condition that can't be controlled or managed except with medication, and (2) Medications taken to control or alleviate symptoms caused by poor lifestyle choices. For example, people take drugs for heartburn, dyspepsia, and acid reflux. These problems are often diet related. Unnecessary use of medication to remedy lifestyle-induced problems results, in part, from the prevailing thought that says it's okay to abuse your body with food or neglect because you can overcome it by swallowing a pill.

Here's a perfect example of socially acceptable abuse: A TV ad for an antacid product depicts a race car driver who must have something to eat after each lap around the track. After the first lap, he eats greasy ribs. After the second lap, he eats greasy fries. For the third lap it's the advertised antacid to the rescue! Fourth lap? He's apparently the winner of the race so there is a huge cake and, yes, more antacid to take care of the cake. Does any of this make sense to you?

Poor health does not have to be part of the aging package. Barring inherited conditions, you can stay in good health not by dependence on medication, but by aggressively and lovingly taking care of yourself. Remember Dr. Rowe's 70-30 ratio. Lifestyle choices matter! I hope that as you read this book, you are reviewing your choices and making new decisions.

Today's drugs are like nothing in the past. Fifty years ago, my father's drug store was a naturalist's delight. Bottles and packages of pharmaceutical-grade roots, leaves, stems, bark, flowers, and berries of plants lined the shelves. My father used those ingredients to make tinctures, syrups, elixirs, and concoctions of every description to treat everything from sore throat to syphilis. I remember a sore throat remedy he made and sold as "Iron Mixture." It was the most vile-tasting stuff you could possibly imagine, but it worked. Were some of those botanicals harmful? Potentially, but doctors and pharmacists knew how and when and in what form to use them safely.

Then, as now, nervousness was a common complaint (we call it stress today) and Elixir of Phenobarbital was the drug of choice to soothe the symptoms. Also then as now, stomach and intestinal complaints were common, but a mixture compounded of three or four herbal ingredients made life bearable. A prescription might have cost a customer $1.50 for a month's supply and they got a refill whenever they asked for it. Whatever did people do without today's high-tech, obscenely expensive antidepressants and proton pump inhibitors? (The latter is a type of stomach medication, not a machine.)

There was just as much to be depressed about (such as World War II), but people learned to cope without medicinal crutches. It wasn't until the appearance of penicillin, followed by more powerful antibiotics, that medication usage began to change. For example, before we had penicillin, when kids got sick with a cold, it just had to run its course with the help of simple remedies to alleviate aches and fever. It didn't take long for that situation to change once doctors started prescribing penicillin to avoid possible "secondary infections" when a child had a cold.

Yesterday's drugs (before penicillin) were relatively benign compared to today's medications which are highly complex, laboratory-engineered substances targeted for specific ailments and often producing an exhaustive list of side effects.

For example, a medication called cimetidine, used to treat stomach problems, also eliminates plantar warts on the bottom of the feet. Think about that. A medication created to target a specific area of the body (stomach) can affect another area of the body in a very unexpected way. It's unnerving. Are there other sleeper side effects of this, or similar drugs now sold over the counter and available to anyone?

Do you pay attention to the side effects rattled off during TV commercials for prescription drugs? You should; it's a real education. Listen carefully to the direct to consumer (DTC) advertising of prescription products. For example, one advertisement says medication designed to alleviate arthritis may cause sudden, unexpected internal bleeding, or liver or kidney damage. Another type of advertised medication declares it may possibly cause flu or ear infections. How could this be? Is anyone listening? How can medicine *cause* flu or an ear infection? A virus causes flu, and bacteria cause infection. The commercials are so cleverly crafted that what remains in the viewer's mind is not the litany of possible horrendous side effects but the powerful visuals, music, and the happiness that depict the promise of relief. Commercials sell an enormous amount of medication. If they didn't, the pharmaceutical companies would not be spending all that money on ad campaigns.

Problems with Multiple Medications

Many consumers experience severe or disturbing side effects from taking multiple medications. This is what happens: You take medication A for arthritis. While alleviating some pain, it causes stomach and intestinal problems. So your doctor prescribes medication B to offset the side effects of medication A. In turn, medication B has side effects of its own. It may cause drowsiness or nausea. You tell the doctor about these side effects and he prescribes medication C to control the drowsiness or nausea. In turn, medication C may create other problems. Before you know it, you may be taking four or more medications. And you wonder why you don't feel well. This is especially a problem with older people in today's HMO world who may see different specialists. It doesn't occur to them to alert each physician to all the medications they take.

Yes, medication is necessary to control diabetes, arthritis, and run-away blood pressure. It helps lower nasty cholesterol and other problems that plague our self-indulgent society, but diet and lifestyle changes can help as much or more.

Yes, medication is necessary to control pain, infection, seizures, and even some condition you were born with or acquired. There are many legitimate uses for medication and we would suffer needlessly without the relief they provide. All medication is not bad. It's the overuse, misuse, and abuse that are bad. Most medications, when taken over an extended period of time, are extremely hard on vital organs such as the liver and kidneys. Prolonged medication use, necessary or not, will seriously impair your ability to put old on hold. Your goal should be to acquire optimum health so, if possible, you won't need a chemical crutch to get you through each day.

The CBC Power Packed Profile

Putting old on hold doesn't start when you reach a particular chronological milestone. It begins right now, whatever your age. One of the best tools you can use to control aging is a comprehensive blood test called the CBC/Chemistry Profile. It's relatively inexpensive and measures 35 blood factors that can have a significant impact on your health. Unfortunately, many HMOs, in an attempt to save money, don't suggest CBC/Chemistry Profiles.

The CBC Profile would help detect problems before they gain a toehold. Even though the Food and Drug Administration (FDA) mandates regular blood testing if you are taking certain medications, doctors often do not order blood tests. This means it's up to you to make sure you are tested. And not just once in your lifetime, but annually or even more frequently. If your doctor won't order a test, or if your insurance won't pay, bite the financial bullet, if possible, and make arrangements on your own. Remember, your health is your responsibility. Outside of California you don't need a physician's order for a blood test. Visit www.YourFutureHealth.com and learn about all the different conditions an appropriate blood test can uncover.

Why is a CBC/Chemistry Profile important? For several reasons:

- Detection of calcium imbalance. If too much calcium leaches from bone and deposits in the vascular system, you may not know it until you suffer a fracture, kidney stone, or heart valve failure due to calcification. Calcium imbalance can be corrected with dietary changes before it becomes a full-blown problem. In this case the CBC/Chemistry Profile can be a lifesaver.
- Detection of high serum glucose, which accelerates development of arterial and neurological conditions. If found in time, you can implement lifestyle changes such as improved nutrition which can also be a lifesaver.
- Detection of excessive amounts of iron, which rampantly generates free radicals that increase the risk of cancer, Alzheimer's, and Parkinson's disease.
- Detection of changes in hormone balance. In both men and women, failure to correct an imbalance can play a role in cardiovascular disease, some types of cancer, Type II diabetes, osteoporosis, depression, abdominal obesity, and reduced physical and mental energy levels.

Typically, most doctors, when treating a woman for menopause, will not do a blood test to determine exactly how much or how little hormone replacement may be necessary, but will automatically prescribe Premarin or other synthetic hormone replacement. The equine conjugated estrogens in Premarin are not equivalent to human female hormones. If your doctor prescribes any kind of hormone without first doing a blood test to determine what or how much you need, insist on it or get one on your own. It's your body and your life. You need to know if you are receiving appropriate treatment. I encourage you to take an active role.

But perhaps the most important reason to have a CBC/Chemistry Profile is to check on how well your liver and kidneys are doing, particularly if you continually take prescription medication. Older people take a lot of medication on a regular basis, some of it unnecessary, and I'm not talking just about those in their sixties and beyond. Boomers take their share of drugs too, and taking regular doses of medication is trending down to ever-younger ages. Adverse reactions to prescription medication contribute to the demise of some 200,000 people per year. That shouldn't happen. If tested often, drug-induced liver and kidney damage could be uncovered before it results in disability or death.

The liver and kidneys are under constant assault, not just from medication but also from toxic substances in the environment and especially from chemical-laden products ingested as "food." I am convinced these two vital organs are not designed to process the wide range of complex and toxic chemicals that assault them on a daily basis. If you read labels and can't pronounce the names of chemical additives in the food products you eat, then just assume your liver and kidneys will have to work overtime to detoxify them. (I had mentioned the importance of reading labels earlier.) Constant stress on these organs eventually takes a toll. Clearly, between prescription medication and faulty diet choices, there is a clear need for annual blood testing. It's up to you to get it done.

Insider Information: Be in the Know

Here's some insider information about medications you might not find elsewhere. I hope this will really get you thinking.

In a pharmacy there are several categories of medications. Here are just a few:

- Antibiotics
- Cholesterol control
- Contraceptives
- Gastric disorder relief
- Pain relief
- Mood alteration
- High blood pressure
- Hormone replacement
- Respiratory relief

On the list above, only one category of medication can produce a cure: Antibiotics. The rest only alleviate or manage symptoms. Think about that. Could diet and lifestyle have a bearing, to some degree or another, on conditions represented in the categories above? Absolutely.

I've mentioned before that customers come to my prescription counter with shopping carts overflowing with the makings of their All-American diet: Manufactured, synthetic, pseudo food, heavy with grease, refined sugar, salt, assorted chemicals, processed, so-called "fresh" meat that may be in an advanced state of putrefaction and bulging with diarrhea-inducing bacteria. Then they pick up prescriptions for high blood pressure, high cholesterol, gastric upset or arthritis pain. With better diet and lifestyle choices, I believe they would need far less medication. What do you think?

Older people trapped in the cycle of food abuse and prescription drug relief may be living longer with the help of their medications, but often they are not living well. I can't count how often I hear the complaint, "I'm taking all of the medication my doctor prescribed, and I still don't feel well." These are old people in every sense of the word. They can't put old on hold. The only thing that's on hold is a visit from the Grim Reaper.

Recently, I read something in a pharmacist's magazine[7] that made me angry. Here are two direct quotations:

"As members of the baby boom generation approach their senior years the retailer is preparing to handle the record number of prescriptions they will certainly require." Will you "certainly require" a record amount of prescription medication as you age? No, you should not, if you start taking care of your health right now.

7 "Retailer ready for aging boomers," *Chain Drug Review*, December 16, 2002 p. 28

The same article stated: "The aging boomers want to remain young and healthier longer, and this will translate into prescription drug therapy to accomplish these goals."

Prescription drug therapy to help remain younger and healthier longer? I think not. Remember, most drug therapy just relieves or manages symptoms and has nothing to do with curing underlying causes of health problems. Are there youth pills out there they are not telling us about? We don't stock any in our pharmacy!

Take care of your health early on and keep it up because clearly, vibrant health does not come out of a prescription bottle. It results from how well you care for yourself over time. It's a test of how much you appreciate and value the one and only body you will ever have.

Retirement

We Need a New Perspective

The face of what we call "old age" is changing. People are living longer and staying in the workforce longer. While more people than ever may be choosing to stay productive, most want to retire and will do so if given the opportunity. With minimal encouragement, it's human nature to want to kick back and do nothing, or do what gives the greatest amount of pleasure. A 2002 U.S. Census Bureau survey showed there were almost 34 million people over age 65 and only 13 percent of them were working or seeking work.

Unless that 13 percent increases significantly we will continue to see typical mental and physical decline attributed to aging: Decline that has little to do with the aging process and a lot to do with effects of retirement. For example, large numbers of retirees are worried and depressed because they must scrape by on insignificant retirement checks. I'm not imagining this. I deal with retirees every day and I know what they are thinking because they tell me. And what they convey to me one way or another is that living on a shoestring is stressful and takes a toll mentally and physically. Knowing the financial, health, and other problems they must struggle with, I can tell you that retirement is not a happy, healthy place to be for anyone who enjoys even marginal mental and physical health.

Retirees are often in denial about what's happening to them. They accept their life the way it is and try to make the best of it. On their best of days they claim they are happy, more or less, free to come and go as they please and yes, maybe they feel they are happy. It's their way of coping. But how happy can one be when there isn't enough money for essentials such as food, medication and vitamins, or for the simple pleasures working people take for granted (vacations and having a few extra dollars to play with). That only 13 percent of people over age 65 work or are looking for work is potentially disastrous. We need to stop pretending that retirement benefits anyone except businesses that profit from retirees, and unscrupulous politicians who pander to the plight of retirees hovering at the poverty level.

The human mind and body are not designed to lie fallow. We simply don't do well when left to our human inclination to do nothing or to pass time with mindless busyness. The old cliché to use it or lose it certainly applies.

Constant admonitions that at age 65 "it's time to stop and smell the roses," or "you've worked hard all your life, now it's time to take it easy," and "you've earned the right to do nothing" fuel the penchant for inactivity. As early as age 50, a relentless cacophony of retirement sound bites emerge from every direction, suggesting that life is almost over and you may as well slow down and prepare for the end. Reaching the mid-century mark legitimizes the release of a barrage of advice and self-serving sales pitches addressing every possible real or imagined need for those of supposedly advanced years.

God bless the ailing and the old. What would corporate America and assorted opportunists do without them? For example, merciless arthritic pain is the focus of drug company TV ads to sell new and expensive prescription drugs with nasty side effects that promise but may not bring relief; the travel industry depends on seniors to sign up to take cruises; financial planners need seniors to buy annuities and other investments; developers of senior communities need retirees to fill their villas; insurance providers need retirees to buy long term care policies; politicians hungry for votes at election time play to impoverished seniors with promises of saving the bankrupt Social Security system; nursing home operators need ailing retirees to fill their beds; gambling casinos lure financially strapped retirees by providing special transportation and low cost meals. One woman actually told me she would rather spend money on gambling than on medication!

Make no mistake. Retirement is big business and a destination of choice for many because it's the traditional and expected thing to do. It's time to rethink this misguided creation of the Depression era. It didn't make sense then and makes even less sense today.

Why Retire?

In my mind, there are just two reasons to retire: You don't want to work or you can't work.

1. You simply don't want to work any more. You are tired of taking orders from some numbskull half as bright as you are. You want to be your own boss and finally do what you want and go where you want when you want. After all, you've worked long and hard and you've earned your retirement. Social custom says it's time. You are ready for the senior lifestyle. Your friends are retired. You want to travel. You'd like to crank up the RV and get on the road with your significant other. The two of you will love being cooped up in that cramped space. Or maybe, you could even take a trip around the world.

You are ready to play Bingo, eat early bird discount dinners, hang out at the senior center, and play cards or shuffleboard with like-minded peers. You want to join the raft of seniors who have all the time in the world to go to casinos and gamble the money they can little afford to lose. Maybe you'd go back to school, and maybe take classes and learn to use a computer. In short, you want your liberation from the daily grind and conformity. What you may not realize is that you will soon move on to another type of structure where you might chafe under the boring, mind numbing conformity often found in the lifestyle of retirees.

2. You retire because you don't have a choice. Your health may have given out and you are unable to continue to work. You may need to take care of ailing parents, even one of your children or grandchildren. Your spouse may require your full attention. Or your employer may find a way to prematurely displace you. Yes, there are

legitimate reasons to retire, and under more favorable circumstances you may have made a different choice.

As I mentioned, I'm a pharmacist by profession. I work full-time in a supermarket pharmacy. I plan to work indefinitely because I don't believe in voluntary retirement, except in certain circumstances. My work is often stressful but always challenging and I value it for these reasons:

- It keeps me sharp and aware, highly youthful characteristics and key elements in putting old on hold. Dealing with the public helps maintain my mental edge and a realistic perspective of the world.
- It inspires me to always look my best. It means I keep up my appearance on a regular basis, not when I feel like it. Regular, systematic maintenance helps me stay ageless. Having a job that motivates me to keep up personal grooming is better than having a mental tape of a nagging mother who keeps harping on me to do what I know I should do.
- It's a great reality check for how I'm doing. I'm at an age when custom and tradition say I should be "slowing down" or "losing my edge." When I work faster and more accurately than a pharmacist 30 to 40 years younger, I know I've put old on hold. It's great for my self-esteem.
- It allows me to help people in ways that would be impossible if I were doing anything else. If I were retired, for example, I would not have exposure to people in

need as I do today. When I think about different lifestyles I could be living, it reinforces my belief that retirement would be a waste of precious time for me, and a loss for others. That's not arrogant; just realistic. I provide a valued service. I provide meaning. Why would I want to give that up?

- It gives me the opportunity to work with some remarkable young people. For an older person, interaction with a young person can be a gift that helps maintain a balanced outlook on life. I'm tempted to say the value of being around young people is not about adopting their behavior, but in some ways they do influence me. In the workplace, for example, mature youngsters are often exquisite teachers of patience, kindness, and extraordinary common sense when dealing with difficult people. More than once, young co-workers have bailed me out of a potentially volatile situation with their unflappable cool, a hallmark of youth I constantly strive to emulate because of its human relations value. They also benefit because I know they are learning some vital lessons about agelessness from working with me.
- It allows me to live relatively stress-free, financially. I don't have to pinch pennies as many seniors do. Working is a blessing and I'm grateful. My heart is heavy for those who exist on Social Security and little else. I feel especially troubled because many poverty-level seniors have the capacity to work. It would undoubtedly ease their financial situation. With the cost of

prescription medication so exorbitant an extra bit of income could make the difference between existing and having a decent quality of life.

- Best of all, my job gives me an intimate, bird's-eye view of the behaviors, thinking, and lifestyles of people of all ages. Sometimes I can't believe I'm paid to do what I do because I learn so much about lifestyles and human nature. For example, I see how many people, rather than change an unwise lifestyle that causes health problems, would rather take a pill with undesirable side effects to control symptoms. I see those of my generation who believe their doctor is God and without question will take as many medications as they are given. Yes, I see and hear a lot and much of it confirms my thinking about the aging process, how it can be better managed, and the importance of positive lifestyle choices. Above all, it reinforces my resolve to keep doing what I'm doing.

Retirement Realities

Okay, you understand your reasons to retire, and some of my reasons not to retire. Now let's look at some retirement realities.

Think about the meaning of the word "retirement." Give it a lot of thought, because it's an extremely powerful word. Ernest Hemingway called it the most depressing word in the English language and I think he was right. Once accepted as a state of being, it can be devastating. Unquestioned acceptance can too quickly lead to resignation.

Think about what retirement really means beyond the golf, travel, gardening or whatever retirees are supposed to find fulfillment in doing. Acceptance and internalization of the word retirement sets into motion a nonstop mental and physical meltdown. Your body may begin to shut down because retirement tells the subconscious you are letting go of life. You go into a holding pattern for the final event. The decline happens so insidiously, so imperceptibly. Deliriously happy retirees in an active state of decline would be the last to realize what is happening to their minds and bodies. A friend or neighbor may quickly spot signs of decline such as slower mental and physical movement, halting speech or changed mental outlook. But retirees would adamantly insist nothing has changed, except that they're happier than they've even been.

When you are not required to deal with what is outside of your comfort zone or wrestle with mental challenges on a daily basis, when you no longer have a goal or dream to strive for, when you live life as merely passing time, then mental and physical decline are inevitable. That's the reality. Use it or lose it is the perfect admonition in this situation.

Here are some retirement realities you'll want to keep in mind:

Retirement Reality No. 1: Loss of Income and Decline in Quality of Life

This is a biggie. Financial gurus say you need 70 percent of your pre-retirement income to live well in retirement yet I can't imagine trying to live on less than my current income. Unexpected expenses can pop up at any time of life, and inevitably, they seem to cost more, and happen more often when you are older. Of course, you can cut back and do without, but where's the fun in that? It could be like starting out in life all over again. Financially, remember how tight things were when you first married and began your career? I do! It was challenging to say the least, and it lasted a long time. Your prime time is not the time to be pinching pennies and depending on special senior benefits to save money so you can meet expenses.

To fully understand the significance of needing an adequate income, I wish you could be in my shoes and see seniors as I do everyday, relying on Social Security. It's heartbreaking. Having $7-$10 to cover the co-pay for medication may not be a big deal when you have sufficient income, but it's tragic when you don't have it and won't have it until the first of the month when your paltry Social Security check arrives. Think about not having $10 in your pocket! As if that's not depressing enough, think about the impoverished seniors existing on Social Security and taking six or more medications each month, and some of those prescriptions cost a good deal more than $10 each. Many seniors on Social Security spend so much money on medication they have little left over for food. Forget about buying vitamins or other diet supplements. That would seem like a luxury to them.

If you want to stay healthy, live reasonably well, and put old on hold, you need money – a lot more than you think, not just for medication but also for quality food and the costly health maintenance that comes with regular use of vitamins and food supplements. I don't care what anybody says, this is not the time of life to even think about cutting back!

Is there a solution? Yes. Many seniors, in spite of health issues, are perfectly capable of working, and they should work as long as it is in keeping with their abilities and preferences. It would keep them in touch with the real world and tremendously boost their self worth, not to mention enhance their quality of life. A financial penalty no longer exists for retirees on Social Security who want to work, so that excuse is no longer valid. It would be wonderful if government or private programs would encourage and prepare healthy retirees, the older the better, to get back into earning a wage. The editor of a senior publication in my area recently lamented, "Every time I have been told a Senior-Back-to-Work program would be set up, it falls through . . . so many qualified seniors are looking for work." Funding is available for so many social programs of questionable worth. Why is it so difficult to get assistance for a program that could radically improve the lives of so many people? Living at the poverty level is the pits when there are alternatives such as finding a job.

California is in the process of making it easier for seniors to find rewarding jobs. A report by University of California's California Policy Research Center[8] has prompted the state Health and Human Services Agency to develop a plan to handle the increase in residents over age 65. Recommendations include offering tax credits to employers who hire and retrain seniors. This won't happen a moment too soon. By the year 2020, California expects to have 6.5 million seniors aged 65 or older compared to 3.5 million in 2001–2002.

8 *San Diego Union Tribune*, April 30, 2001 p. A3

Retirement Reality No. 2: Difficulty Going Back to Work

If you retire for even a brief period, then decide retirement isn't for you and you try to go back to your former line of work, it may be difficult if you haven't kept your skills current. It doesn't take long to lose your mental and physical edge. I have seen this happen with pharmacists who can't wait to get out of the business. The long hours and stress of dealing with the public eventually take a toll. After six months or a year away from the daily grind, they decide they are bored or need money and go back to work. Yet the person who retired six months or a year ago is no longer the same person. In that short period of time a person's mental and physical agility can become impaired. Speech, movement, reaction time, and the ability to learn have lessened. Plain and simple, the sharpness has dulled. These individuals are still competent, but their inner light is no longer shining brightly, just flickering. The edge is gone and is sometimes difficult to resurrect. Not impossible, but difficult. Some pharmacists, recognizing their retirement-induced deficiencies, give up and retreat back into inactivity. It's a great loss of experience, ability and knowledge.

I suggest staying employed as long as possible. Keep up your skills. The bridge from the real world to retirement is short, alluring, and convenient. If you retire and decide to take the road back, you may find it rocky at best or impassable at worst. Of course, if you are lucky, you may reach a fork in the road that will lead you to a new and exciting place.

Does this mean you should never take a vacation from work? Not at all. It's important to give your mind, body and spirit the opportunity to rest and rejuvenate. Periodically you need time away from everyday concerns to think, let go of unproductive stress, and allow your brain to process budding ideas and clarify goals. Just be certain you understand the difference between a sabbatical and a "slide into retirement." You are on vacation when you know you are returning to something fulfilling, challenging and productive, something you eagerly look forward to tackling.

Sliding into retirement is deceptively easy. It occurs when you tell yourself you are just enjoying an extended vacation, taking time to stop and smell the roses. You revel in that intoxicating scent of freedom and inhale so deeply of the sweetness that you drift into a state of mindless inebriation. Before you know where time went, no longer do you smell the roses; you are pushing up daisies. Your tombstone reads: "Mary Jones: She stopped so long to smell the roses, she neglected to pursue her dreams and reach her potential. Her greatness is interred here with her remains." Rest (but not too long) and restore yourself, then get on with living, and working, and being productive. Fulfill your dreams and develop your innate gifts as long as you live. It's too exciting an adventure to forfeit simply because of chronological age.

Retirement Reality No. 3:
Loss of Self Esteem and Personal Power

Many seniors suffer from depression. I am convinced depression often results from a loss, major change, repressed anger or painful life event. Those are not the only causes, but retirement, no matter how much you may look forward to it, is a major transition, often a traumatic event. It's closure on a lifetime of contribution. It's saying goodbye to part of you that will never exist again, except in memory. It can be no less devastating than the death of a loved one.

One day you have a title and a recognizable value in our society. The next day you retire and now the word retired precedes the title and distinction you enjoyed for so many years. Your value to society has instantly diminished and so has your status. You've gone from being a somebody to a nobody. How often have you heard it said of someone, "Didn't he used to be a lawyer," or "Wasn't she a surgeon at one time?" or "Wasn't that person a physicist?" Regardless of what they used to be, they are all now retired and, like it or not, the expectation of being less valuable or competent will hover over them as long as they live. These social assumptions influence the way retirees see themselves, and the way others see and treat them.

Some time ago, I had a conversation with an 81-year-old man who works as an investment consultant. Speaking with him on the phone, I would never guess his age. His voice was strong and youthfully masculine, and he expressed himself quickly and clearly. His views on the downside of retirement confirmed some of my thinking. He believed retirement could be particularly difficult for a man who, pre-retirement, held a managerial or other powerful position. One day he is behind a desk giving orders and receiving deferential treatment and respect. The day after he retires, it's all over.

A lifetime of defining his identity in his work is gone. And it's gone for good. If he is married, he is now taking orders from a new boss, a wife who likely has been in charge of things on the home front and holds seniority in domestic management decisions. She has her daytime lifestyle and he had his. Now, he's living *her* lifestyle, like it or not.

If he gets bored, he can accompany his wife on shopping trips to the supermarket and drive her crazy urging her to hurry up or questioning her selections. That she has successfully run the home and planned meals without his help for the past umpteen years never occurs to him. Or maybe he can tag along when she has a yen to cruise around the mall, and he can cool his heels while she tries on clothes in one department store after another. We've all seen the old guys at malls huddled together on benches, looking dour and impatient while wives or girlfriends shop till they drop. Or maybe he can have fun sitting in on his wife's bridge games, dishing the dirt with the girls. Small wonder that retirement can create major friction in a marriage previously considered harmonious.

No doubt about it: After you retire your value as a human being and your professional or business abilities immediately diminish in the eyes of the world. You may know in your heart of hearts that you are still the same capable person, but the general negative disregard and feedback does terrible things to your self-esteem.

Does that make you uncomfortable? It should! The subconscious understands the word retirement to mean closing the door on life. In the state of retirement, focusing on the past and without life-affirming goals for the future, you are helping to create that lackluster reality. Each day gets closer to the inevitable and that's enough to make anyone feel depressed.

There are ways of making retirement fulfilling, productive and meaningful. How about doing volunteer work? Many worthwhile causes and institutions could not function without unpaid help, and for them volunteer work is vital. However, I don't encourage volunteer work as a primary retirement activity because, frankly, I have mixed feelings about seniors working gratis unless they are living above the poverty level. If you are struggling financially (as so many are), and are capable of productive work, I encourage you to seek a paying job. However, before looking for a job that pays decently, it's essential to become computer literate. It's not difficult to find computer classes for beginners. Most local schools and community colleges offer them. After you become even minimally techno-savvy, all kinds of opportunities will open up. If you had a pre-retirement job that paid very well be realistic about what salary you will now accept.

I have a friend who does volunteer work several days a week. She's only marginally secure financially so I asked why she volunteers instead of having a paying job. She said she would like extra income but because of her age, she doesn't feel very qualified to hold a paying job. As a volunteer she feels she works on her terms, which is not entirely true; they wouldn't rely on her as they do if she didn't produce. Because she's been doing the same volunteer work for years, she's as competent as one could ask. How heartbreaking that she has so little faith in her ability simply because of her age.

It warms the heart and soul to freely help others and expect nothing in return. Such kindness should be encouraged, yet, there is magic in receiving a paycheck for work well done. It is liberating both financially and emotionally; it boosts self-esteem as little else can, particularly at a time in life when self-sufficiency is not expected or encouraged.

Retirement Reality No. 4: Adopting the Senior Lifestyle

Without question, opportunities to expand your world can come with retirement if you are healthy enough to travel, or go back to school and you can afford the expense. Many people are happy staying active and engaged, without being particularly productive or challenged. They are living life passively. If that makes them happy, fine, but I'll choose active over passive any day.

In my experience, many retirees (not all) live in a narrow, sheltered world in which they see the same people and do the same things every day. They stay close to home, venturing out to go shopping, to the doctor, or to church. There is little if any challenge to keep their intellect fired up. They sit passively in front of a TV most of the day, unaware the brain and body are turning to mush. They find it difficult to keep up with change.

I recall a retired woman on antidepressant medication complaining the world was moving so fast, and she couldn't keep up with everything, particularly computers. It made her feel left behind and this bothered her terribly. Don't allow yourself to get to such a state. Welcome change, and embrace it. A good way is to stay in touch with young people who thrive on change. You can emulate coping techniques that work for them. It will help you put old on hold.

Another aspect of the senior lifestyle is the tendency to fall into a group mentality. Just as teens associate in packs to establish their identity, define their lifestyle, and find emotional support, many seniors become similarly peer dependent. They refer to themselves and their friends as "us old people" and take a perverse pride in inviting sympathy, playing up feebleness, describing symptoms and using deprecating terms to describe their age, circumstances, or abilities. Personal identity, individuality and independence are lost to group decisions, attitudes and activities. This observation certainly does not apply to all old people, but I see enough of this on a daily basis to view it with alarm.

I've also witnessed an irrational group entitlement mentality. For example, at the onset of flu season in the fall of 2000, it became evident flu vaccine was in short supply and scheduled shots had to be canceled. Most people accepted the situation, but some were irate. One woman complained, "But I'm a senior citizen, we're supposed to get those shots before anybody else." Be on guard for unreasonable self-absorption. Whiney, complaining victims forfeit agelessness. Clearly, not all old people exhibit this type of behavior, but enough of them do. I encourage you to constantly monitor your mindset as you age.

While we're on the subject of narrowing your world and regressing to group-dependent behavior, let's explore the retirement community phenomenon, the ultimate resurgence of the adolescent group mentality.

Most people living in retirement communities are happy and content. They wouldn't live any place else and that's fine.

But I consider that this is an unnatural segregated environment, locked away and separated from young people, isolated from people unlike themselves. Surrounded by gates, guards, walls, security cameras, perfectly manicured, sterile lawns, topiary, sculptures, waterfalls, and ponds complete with ethereal white swans, retirement communities often seem like a hybrid of a minimum-security prison and a cemetery. I have friends who moved into a retirement community believing it would be utopian. They quickly discovered that lifestyle wasn't for them. Of course, these friends were independent types and should have known better. But then, they weren't expecting regimentation and stifling structure, they just expected a nice life.

Retirement Reality No. 5: Unproductive Use of Time

Philosopher and mathematician Bertrand Russell observed the importance of work in his book, *The Conquest of Happiness,* where he states, "Most people, when they are left free to fill their own time according to their own choice, are at a loss to think of anything sufficiently pleasant to be worth doing . . . To be able to fill leisure time intelligently is the last product of civilization, and at present, very few people have reached this level."[9]

I witness this truth every day. It's not the people who are working hard and trying to make ends meet who usually end up miserable. It's those with so much time on their hands that

9 Russell, Bertrand, *The Conquest of Happiness,* Chapter 14 page 162

they can focus on minor annoyances and inconveniences in their lives.

Here's an example: Because so many seniors are in dire financial straights, they spend a good deal of time figuring out how to get the most for their money. This is good, but in the process they can dominate a merchant's time asking why this item is priced $2.00 higher than a competitor's is. A retiree recently accosted me with that question. I told him I honestly didn't know why our price was $2.00 higher; that was a corporate decision. In most pharmacies, prices are computer generated; I have no control over how they are determined. He didn't seem to understand my explanation so he persisted, saying, "Well, why don't you know? It's your job to know." I was at a loss so I gave him an 800 number to call for a more satisfactory answer. Apparently, the 800 number didn't work out and he was back the next day, asking for a name and address to which he could direct his question. I can look at this situation two ways: Much ado about nothing or bully for him. Retirees who are still capable of productivity and keeping meaning in their lives are able to respond with positive action instead of complaints when challenges arise. After all, it's the people with time on their hands who can focus on minor troubles in their lives. Perhaps taking on this problem and addressing it made him feel productive. And considering how little Social Security provides, I can appreciate that $2.00 may seem significant.

Here's another example of much ado about nothing: We were living in an enclave of townhouses originally built for occupants 18 and older. There were no walls, gates, or guards; it was just a restricted development in one section of town. Stringent community regulations mandated that pet owners must clean up after their pets. At the time, we had a little cockapoodle named Samantha that weighed about 10 pounds dripping wet. Being conscientious pet owners and wanting to be good neighbors, when we walked our little darling, we always carried a bag and scooper, wanting to do our part to keep the community in the required pristine condition.

I recall three incidents that gave credence to Bertrand Russell's observation about having too much time to fuss about minor annoyances. On one occasion, after our little dog left a little pile on someone's lawn, we dutifully picked it up. As we walked away, an elderly man opened a window and yelled, "Stop that! It leaves a terrible smell behind!" What were we to do? We had completely cleaned up the mess. We amused ourselves thinking that on future outings we would carry a can of disinfectant spray and spritz the offending area after picking up. After all, we wanted to be good neighbors.

Another time our little darling took a particularly long time to urinate. When she finally decided she was done and we started to walk away, a woman flung open her door and screamed, "Go back and pick it up!" Well, there was nothing to pick up. It had already seeped into the ground.

Once, as we were walking past a neighbor, Samantha stopped to leave a few drops. The neighbor whom we had greeted with a cheery hello now glared at us and snarled, "Your dog is staining the grass!" Indeed, some people need to be busier!

I relate these stories as encouragement to monitor your thinking, behavior, and emotional state closely as the years roll by. Now, while you still have your wits about you, resolve to constantly stay aware of your conduct and mental outlook, and notice how it may be changing over time. As a reality check, evaluate how your social performance stacks up against that of young people. The purpose is to emulate not their immaturity but their spontaneity and ability to stay flexible. Your behavior will take care of itself if you continue to remain in the real world, physically, mentally, and emotionally. It will help you maintain your self-respect and sensitivity to the feelings of others, and will definitely help you put old on hold

I can immediately distinguish a completely retired senior from one who is still working, even part-time. The difference is like day and night. The person still involved with the realities of life is much more reasonable and easier to deal with. That person is successfully managing the aging process while the other is listing toward the ultimate outcome. Why get old before your time?

Having made some negative comments and observations about retirement and retirees, I acknowledge many retired people are happy with their lifestyles. They are content and not crotchety; they consider their lives full and even overflowing with activity. There aren't enough hours in the day to do shopping, taking care of the home, cooking, attending classes, gardening, vacationing, golfing, and visiting the doctor. Those blissful people are entitled to do what they want and no one would want to take any of their happiness away from them. They find comfort and satisfaction in the structure and sameness of a day-to-day routine. Indeed, happiness, like beauty, is in the eye and experience of the beholder.

Yet, as I see it, those happy folks are not putting old on hold because that concept is beyond their comprehension or interest. They see themselves as old people and that defines how they now live and look at the world. They are going with the flow, doing what they believe they should be doing at their age and they have a good deal of company to prove they are in the right groove.

Alternative to Retirement: Seamless Living

So what I'm saying is that retirement is not the way to go if you want to put old on hold. And you may be asking, what's the alternative?

Simple. *Plan to live seamlessly.* Think about those four words. Plan. To live. Seamlessly. Those words mean exactly what they say.

If you want to be victorious over the aging process it's not going to happen because you think it would be a good idea. Putting old on hold is possible only if you believe it can be done, and you have a plan and a commitment to make that plan a reality. It's not a lot of work; it's not that difficult. It just requires your ongoing attention. And that plan must include preparation for you to live productively and seamlessly in continuous growth, without self-inflicted traumatic breaks (such as retirement), that can impair your vitality, your mind, your health, and how you live your life.

Your Bolt of Life

Think of your life as a bolt of beautiful red satin cloth, unfolding seamlessly before you. Satin allows you to shape and drape the fabric however you like. Imagine there are approximately 100 yards on the bolt. You don't know for sure the actual number of yards because there isn't an accurate way to determine the length just by looking at it. In that respect, this bolt of fabric is like life. You just don't know when or where the end is. Let's unfurl the cloth 10 yards at a time and assign each 10 yards a decade of your life. This reveals the way your life unfolds:

- From birth to age 20, you are getting set up for life. At age 20, you are in school preparing for a specific career or starting out in a job that will launch one of several careers. You don't think about your health; you know you are invincible. You trash your body and get away with it, but not for long. Time is marching on and is catching up with you, sight unseen.
- At age 30, you are involved in your career, perhaps in a relationship, buying a home, or married and maybe starting a family. From a health standpoint you begin to realize there are limits to how much you can abuse your body and you begin to see little signs of aging.
- At age 40, you are advancing in your career and raising kids. You begin to notice softness in the jaw, belly, thighs, and backside. Things are beginning to slip and slump! So far, you've opened out 40 yards of material representing the length of life you've lived so far. It's

gone; you can't get it back, and probably wouldn't want to. I hope you've grown in wisdom and maturity during those 40 years because you are going to need those virtues later on. You are beginning to think of yourself as middle aged, probably because health problems are becoming evident. Back stiffness and joint discomfort appear without warning letting you know arthritis may be around the corner.

- At age 50, things begin to change dramatically. Life (being alive, staying alive) becomes more serious. Health challenges that began in your forties are not letting up. More stiffness and joint pain, and aches and odd feelings you never experienced before pop up unexpectedly. Not only will you deal with more health issues, you will now confront another situation: The marketers just waiting for you to turn 50 because they have a lot to sell you in preparation for your "final years."

Here are five things sure to occur when you reach age 50, all suggesting the end is near:

- You receive an invitation to join AARP. When that happens, you will return the solicitation unopened, marked "return to sender," thinking there is nothing wrong with AARP, but you're not ready yet. Maybe you'll consider joining later on.
- Real estate agents will call, wanting to sell you a retirement villa in Heavenly Hills, the land of the living

dead. After all, it's a given you will retire and, surely, you will want to spend your last days with people like you.

- Insurance agents will try to sell you a policy for your final expenses. You certainly don't want your loved ones left financially holding the bag, (or coffin), as the case may be.
- Financial planners call during your dinner hour, wanting to sell you a great annuity so you'll have a comfortable retirement.
- But you know it's all over when the sweet young thing who takes your order for coffee and a greasy burger at the fast food emporium scrutinizes your wrinkles and asks, "Will that be senior coffee, ma'am?" It's worse yet if she just assumes you are over the hill and gives you a senior coffee discount without asking if you want it.

Preparing for Your Second Life

Pay no attention to those who imply your life will soon be over just because you've hit fifty. It's not over. Far from it. Instead of listening to death and decrepitude mongers, get your defiant attitude in gear and begin taking these steps:

- If you haven't done so already, this is your last chance to get serious about taking responsibility for optimizing your health. You are only 50 or thereabouts, and even if you are older, much older, remember how incredibly forgiving your body can be once you decide to start treating it right. But don't put off this decision any longer.

- Develop a plan to stay productive for the rest of your life. That may mean saving like crazy to start your own business so that when your current employer shows you the door at age 65, you can smile in anticipation of the beginning of your second life. Yes, financial planning is crucial for future success, but instead of calling it retirement planning, call it future planning, or second life planning. Words have power! If you persist in using the term "retirement planning," you may not save as much as you could because of the negative connotation of the word "retirement" or the misguided expectation that somehow, Social Security will help.
- Your plan may include going back to school full-time for an advanced degree or training for the career of your dreams. Ridiculous? Only if you've been listening to naysayers who tell you it's impossible or is a waste of time. Remember, chronological age doesn't matter. Look at the late life accomplishments of Colonel Sanders, or Grandma Moses. Look at newsman Mike Wallace, now over 80 and still going strong. Look at it this way. If at age 65 you go back to school, spend five years in classes, and stay in excellent health to age 95 or 100 or more, will it have been wasted time? Of course not. You will have had 25 or more years to improve the quality of your life and, probably, the lives of countless others.

If you think all of this is pie-in-the-sky stuff, or you are not convinced of its soundness, think about this: The California Policy Research Center report dealing with the anticipated increase of Californians over age 65 recommends providing college scholarships to help older Californians prepare for new careers. With this exciting information, I rest my case.

It's selfish to hide your ageless abilities or leave your potential untapped. Get them out there. Let your talent make the world a better place. Believe me, age 50 is not a harbinger of death or even slowing down. It's an opportunity to look forward to the best years of your life, an unprecedented second life.

Back to the bolt of red satin: You've lived another 10 years so let's unwind another 10 yards. Here you are at age 60, getting ready to rock and roll because, for the past 10 years, you have been preparing eagerly and joyfully for the next exciting phase of your life.

You will thumb your nose at tradition that says it's time to retire. You will not cave in to custom and cut the cloth, saying, "This is all the life I want to live productively." You don't know how many yards of cloth remain on the bolt and you really don't care. You are ready to go on, seamlessly, and without trauma, building, growing, and living fully, unconcerned about the number of years you may have left. You have drafted your will and made other appropriate legal preparations. You are going to get on with living as if you will live forever. You will ignore the numbers. You will *LIVE* your life fully and fabulously: *ALL OF IT*!

If you still think retirement may be the right thing for you but you'd like a second opinion, in the Resources section you'll find Dr. Donald R. Germann's *Retirement is Over-Rated*. He's a seventy-something radiologist, who more than once decided retirement was not for him. He went back to work.

His story will motivate and inspire you. He'll answer many insider questions you've always wanted to ask about health care costs and Social Security. He is candid and down-to-earth; writing in an engaging, easy-to-read style.

Remember, the human mind and body maintains integrity and health when it is engaged in challenging, valuable activity and goal-oriented behavior. It helps to remain accountable to someone or something outside yourself, regardless of your age.

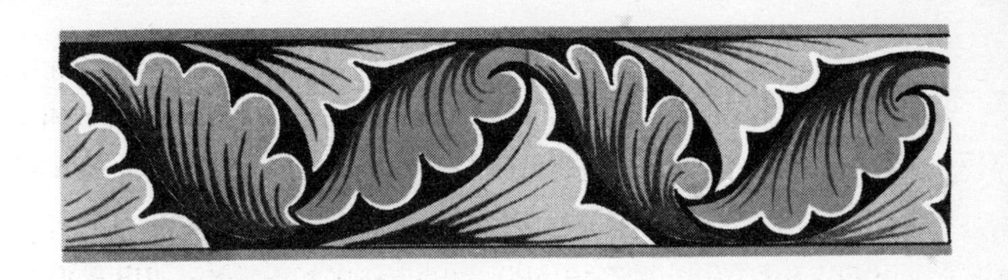

Attitude

Agelessness Begins with Attitude

Attitude is everything. It's a cliché we've heard so often we hardly pay attention when we hear it. I encourage you to pay attention because, attitude *is* everything. Repeat that phrase over and over until it becomes a mantra; an essential part of your daily approach to living. During the day when you know you are cranky or impatient, remind yourself that your behavior is entirely your choice. Just as you choose how to respond to an irritating person or a nasty situation, you can also choose how you will respond to the aging process.

What is your attitude about aging? In particular, what's your attitude about how *you* are aging? Are you aware of the changes you are experiencing over time? If not, you will never be able to take steps to prevent the loss of youthful attributes. It begins with awareness. If you are not aware of your subtle mental and physical changes, you are giving up without a fight: You are relinquishing your personal power. You are letting life happen on its terms, not yours.

Here's what I mean: Think of youth as a beautiful silver vase, a gift you received at birth. When it's new, your vase is shiny and gleaming without imperfections. However, if you don't take care of the precious vase as the years go by, tarnish will build up when you aren't looking. Of course, you can restore the shine, but you know it will take some effort, and what's a little tarnish, anyway? It's easy to let something more important or more fun take precedence. "I'll polish it next week," you might say, but next week never comes. Do you know anyone who takes time to polish anything anymore?

Well, it's the same with your body. One day, you look in the mirror and see a reflection you've never seen before. It can't be the same body you've been living in all these years, or is it? Yes, it is your body and it's tarnished, big time! You move closer to the mirror to be certain you see what you think you see. Up close, it's even worse. Not only do you see your image, such as it is, you may see a semblance of your mother or father. Egad! You shake your head in horror and exclaim, "Oh my goodness, I look terrible. How did this happen, and when?" It happened because gradualism did its work. You didn't pay attention to how you were changing. Yes, you are wearing clothes a couple of sizes larger, but you didn't realize how far things had gone. If you had remained aware and vigilant, you would not have allowed the pounds to pile up. You would not have given in to buying a larger size; you would have put a stop to the weight gain while it was still controllable.

But that's past history. Now you are outraged and determined to get back into fighting form. You sign up at a fitness center, but after three months of grunting, groaning, sweating, and living on a crash diet, you realize how much work it is and you give up. You rationalize your decision by stating that you don't have the time or energy to become the slim sylph you used to be. You resign yourself to accepting what you have become. And the downward spiral into decline continues. The tarnish gets darker and denser and eventually old age gets the upper hand.

Don't allow the tarnish to build up. Take stock of the youthful characteristics you have at whatever age you are right now. Restore what you can and maintain it constantly. Do not put off maintenance. It's completely doable, and it's well worth the effort. Remember, aging is not like a TV mini-series that's over in five nights. It goes on for the duration. You're living longer, and your life won't be prime time unless you are in prime condition. You can do it!

Not too long ago, age 65 was as long as people lived. That anyone could live to 85 was considered amazing. In the past century, the American lifespan has lengthened by 27 years. There are now more centenarians than ever, and their numbers continue to increase. Isn't that exciting? What will you do with your bonus years? What will they be like? Do you see yourself locked away in a nursing home, dependent on others for your care, or will you be healthy, independent and productive?

Will 100 be the maximum number of years you can expect to live? I don't think so. If age 65 was the norm just a few short decades ago, 100 or more could become the norm in the near future. Consider this: In California alone, the number of those aged 85 and older will increase 200 percent in the next 40 years. Very likely, you too, will benefit from this exciting longevity phenomenon. Even if 100 becomes the norm, I believe accepting *any* number as the maximum number of years you can expect to live places limitations on planning, achievement, and quality of life.

Avoid Limitation Thinking

Many older people don't begin new projects with a long time line because they think, "Maybe I'll never see the fruit of my labors. I just can't justify the time or expense of getting started on something I'll never finish." So instead of embarking on an exciting, challenging, longevity-enhancing project, they sit in their rocking chairs, complaining there is nothing worthwhile to do, feeling sorry for themselves and lamenting how little they've gotten out of life. They just wait for the Grim Reaper to come calling. You, of course, are not going to do that.

To help bolster your resolve to stay in the game for keeps here are some inspirational examples of how it's never too late:

- James Russell Wiggins, at 95, is editor of the *Ellsworth American*, a weekly newspaper in Ellsworth, Maine. What a guy. He thinks retirement is a waste of labor and talent. To him, it's alarming to see people in their sixties, in full possession of their faculties, lolling around retirement communities, giving in to lassitude. "How can society support such idleness?" he laments. (*Los Angeles Times*, May 5, 1999)
- Sadie Lynette, 91, owns Lynette Antiques, a 1400 square-foot shop she runs by herself in Long Beach,

California. She works four to five days a week, seven hours a day, and does all her own bookkeeping. The shop has been in operation for 26 years and she takes pride in doing business the old-fashioned way, which she considers a secret of her success. If a customer isn't satisfied with a purchase, she offers a refund or exchange. She says working keeps her healthy and she chides the old ladies who waste time watching TV all day long. She takes a variety of vitamins even though doctors don't approve, and is convinced supplements are responsible for her good health and longevity. She does her own cooking, shopping and housekeeping. She has given up driving and relies on a loving grandson to take her to work and bring her home every day. Her children are of retirement age but remain active, chips off the old block. Sadie is an absolute inspiration. If I didn't know her age, I'd never guess. Her voice is strong, youthful, and clear; her thoughts and words come without hesitation. There is nothing old about Sadie. Her mental and speech acuity are consistent hallmarks of older people who stay challenged and productive.

- At 82, radio legend Paul Harvey signed a 10-year, $100 million contract with ABC. Why would ABC make such a "foolish" gamble? Harvey claims he lied about his age. "I told them I was 55." His doctor confirmed his excellent health and authorized him to become an astronaut. Why would Harvey want to commit himself to another 10 years of what he has done for the past 50 years? He jokes, "I'd hate to get up every morning to play golf, the way I play golf." As for retirement, it's out of the question[10]. Work is keeping Harvey young, and to look at him and listen to him, that's obvious.

- Some time ago, I interviewed Cliff Holliday, a gentleman who, at 100, goes to work every day solving problems for seniors at the California Congress of Seniors in Los Angeles. I didn't meet him in person but in speaking with him on the phone, I'd never have guessed he was 100. His voice is strong and vibrant. He speaks clearly and quickly, and he attributes his youthfulness to going to work every day. It is not uncommon for him to work until midnight, then get up early and take the bus to work. What an inspiring role model! It made me feel so good to talk to him. He gave me hope for my ability to stay productive at an advanced age.
- A personal friend is 80, but you'd never believe it to look at or speak with him. He creates unique miniature model trains, and there is nothing like it on the market. As he perfects his project he's looking for financial backing to start a new company so he can market his product. Remember, he's 80 and is challenged with some significant health problems. But that doesn't keep him from planning for the future. He is putting old on hold in a big way. What an inspiration.

In an average month, 3.7 percent of people age 90 or above, or at least 50,000 people are in the U.S. workforce[11].

10 *Fortune*, December 18, 2000
11 *Los Angeles Times*, May 5, 1999

That's awesome. Not too many years ago, this was unheard of. People just didn't live that long and, if they did, they didn't work. They were incarcerated in nursing homes or confined to wheelchairs, frail, and barely clinging on to life.

The American Medical Association has identified at least 1,200 physicians age 90 and above who still see patients. And why shouldn't they if they can still provide quality care? Their mental, physical and professional proficiency does not hinge on a chronological number. If they can keep up their skills by engaging in mandatory continuing education and stay current with new developments, that is what counts.

Whatever you do, please do not engage in limitation thinking. Reject negative, flat-earth thoughts. Regardless of your chronological age, fulfill your dreams to the best of your ability. You may surprise yourself and achieve far more than anything you could imagine. In fact, you might achieve one set of far flung goals and then create another.

Appreciate and Associate with Younger People

Limiting social contact to those of your own age hastens decline. Becoming isolated and insulated in a seniors only enclave or otherwise avoiding interaction with younger people is a sure-fire way to prematurely slide into old age. Senior communities are popular but I'm not sure they provide the healthiest way to live. You tend to emulate the thinking and behavior of those you associate with most often, and if you regularly socialize with people who look, think, and act old, you will tend to behave like them.

You'll stay younger by spending time with younger people. Everyone benefits from the energy, excitement, optimism, and, yes, the immaturity of youth. Indeed, that same enthusiasm can be obnoxious at times, maybe even a good share of the time but so is the entitlement attitude of older people. You would agree with this if you dealt with old people who deliberately yank you around and get in your face. I'll never forget the old fellow who was a deliberate, calculated nuisance.

Here's a typical encounter with him: One day he was trying to get his prescription filled using an expired insurance card. He knew it was inactive but he wanted to use it because he thought the co-pay on his new insurance was higher. Finally agreeing that his old insurance no longer existed, he reluctantly pulled out his new card. To his delight and surprise, his new plan didn't have a co-pay at all. That's when he said, "Aren't us old people a pain in the neck?" Yes, old people like him can be a pain in the neck.

Surely, young people can be just as wily, but at least they don't blame it on their youth. Frankly, I'd rather be around young people with a fresh, outrageous outlook on life than around old people consumed with bitterness and remorse who are out of touch with reality. Young people give hope and promise that there is a fulfilling future for everybody. And they need us as mentors. Their floundering and immaturity beg for mature adults to guide them with wisdom, experience, and love. When you provide this guidance, you're better for it and so are they.

Trust Your Ability

While some elderly people become more demanding, others lose the courage to stand on their own two feet. Instead, they expect others to do for them what they could do for themselves. One of my customers, a little old lady (yes, she describes herself that way) is sharp as a tack, but she never shops without a friend (who is almost as old as she is) to help her write checks. She complains that financial transactions make her nervous and her hand wobbles. I've observed nothing wrong with her writing or her hands, but she takes pride in having someone do things for her. Obviously, she has given up her ability to put old on hold.

By law, all medications dispensed by a pharmacy must have childproof caps. If customers want an easy-off cap they can sign a form absolving the pharmacy of liability if the container gets in the hands of a child and causes a problem. Many customers complain, saying the childproof caps are difficult to get off, but like most things, it's easy when you know what to do. "I don't have the strength," is a common complaint. "I have to ask my grandchildren to help me."

If you can lift a fork, you can manage a childproof cap. I will make an allowance for weak, frail individuals, or those with advanced arthritis in their hands – but if you are neither weak nor frail, decide right now that childproof caps will not annoy you today or in the future. It's a choice. Here's how to deal with the inconvenience: Just hold the bottle in one hand and, with the other hand, simultaneously press down on the cap and turn it counter clockwise. Voila, it's off. Practice makes perfect. Even though I demonstrate how easy it is, many people, including big strong men, resist being self-sufficient. "Don't bother to show me how to do it. Just give me an easy-off cap," they say. If that bottle were filled with chocolate or some other tasty ingestible, or a nugget of gold, I wonder how many people would find it difficult.

As you age, please do not allow loving family and friends to suggest "you don't have to do that anymore; we'll do it for you." They may mean well and it's tempting to let others do for you. But if you can do things for yourself, thank them for their concern and, with all the kindness you can muster, let them know you are not senile and can still take care of yourself. If you stay strong you demonstrate that when they reach your age, they can and should be tough and independent, too. Killing loved ones with kindness begins as early as age fifty. It's not because they think of you as particularly needy; their offers of help are born of love and concern and a sense that "it's our turn to take care of you."

A lot of the "we'll do for you" attitude is part of tradition. In the "old country" it's often a given that younger family members will take care of their elders. In our culture, sometimes it's expected and carried out, but increasingly, as younger family members have burdensome obligations, this practice is disappearing.

I recall listening to a talk show when a young mom called to ask for help with her 73-year-old grandmother who lived with the young mom's parents. The problem was that the caller's parents worked, and on weekends, they liked to get away but often found it impossible because perfectly healthy grandma did not like to be left alone.

Grandma had the attitude that all of her life she had taken care of others and now it was time for others to take care of her. This woman's needless dependence and sense of entitlement was causing so much dissention in the family that young mom's parents wanted to put grandma in a nursing home. Of course, grandma resisted. It's nice when we can all get what we want but that's not the real world. Be appreciative if loving family members want to do for you, but resist and avoid contrived dependence as you age. Adult children have problems of their own. They don't need parent-turned-child to add to their burdens.

Unnecessary dependence-inducing help will hasten decline and eventually lead to friction, blame and resentment. Nobody wins. Take pride in accepting responsibility for yourself and trusting your abilities. It will enhance your ability to put old on hold.

Twenty Rules to Get It All Together

There are many ways to get it all together to achieve agelessness. Here are 20 rules to help you do it. In one way or another they are all about having a can-do attitude.

Exercise!

Exercise is essential, but honestly, I find it boring. I would rather do anything else. But, guess what? When I get home from work (about 9:30 in the evening), one of the first things I do is jump on the treadmill and walk for 30 minutes. No self-talk about how tired I am; no rationalization that I have to get up early tomorrow; no mental discussion of any kind. I know why I must do it, so I do it.

If exercise is difficult for you, how about simple stretching? Are you old enough to remember the Romper Room TV show for kids? Remember how the always smiling teacher, Miss Nancy, (or whatever they called her in your area) encouraged her young charges to bend and stretch, and reach for the moon? You can do it too. How about parking your car a distance from work or shops and walk? Early morning mall walking is popular – cool in summer and warm in winter. Use stairs for one or two floors instead of elevators. Just avoid being sedentary! Not only will you do yourself a favor from a health standpoint; when you are in "babe condition" you will look great in your clothes (or without them, too).

Even though the importance of exercise is common knowledge, some women are afraid to work out. Dr. Sandra O'Brien Cousins, a professor of Physical Education and Recreation at the University of Alberta[12], surveyed more than 300 women over the age of 70 about the benefits and risks of fitness activities. Respondents recognized the benefits of exercise but had strong reservations. Comments included, "My heart would hemorrhage," "My muscles would seize up," and "They would carry me out on a stretcher." Some flat-out feared death as a risk of exercising.

Recently I met Stella, a stunning, slim woman in her late fifties. In our discussion about successful aging, she said although she exercised and was in excellent physical condition, she was careful not to do anything that might cause

12 Womansage.com 10-2000

injury. For example, the last time she cleaned windows (the lift-out kind), they seemed terribly heavy and she decided that would be the last time she would tackle that chore. Personally, I don't blame her for not wanting to clean windows ever again. Why bother? It's a thankless job because they just get dirty again. Long ago I decided I would not waste one more moment of my life doing windows and it turned out to be one of my more prudent domestic management decisions! Have you ever seen a goddess wash a window? Not around here you won't!

But even as I understand Stella's desire not to injure herself (certainly a legitimate concern) I wonder if she has the best attitude. She could have said, "I need to do more strength training. There is no reason why this job should be any more difficult than it used to be." Part of the secret to putting off getting old is staying aware of how you are changing over time, and doing what you can to stop or reverse decline while you still can.

I've made a decision to stay strong every way I possibly can. On the days I don't work late, I lift weights in addition to walking on the treadmill. Walking at a fast pace enables me to move quickly and with assurance. Walking and weight training are two ways I avoid osteoporosis. In addition, yoga, which I began in my thirties, helps maintain a high level of physical flexibility.

When I see people my age tottering unsurely and leaning on a cane, I think it is so unfortunate. A labored, uncertain step indicates decline and old age, a conclusion confirmed in a survey of 200 people whose ages ranged from 18 to 80 years of age[13]. Only seven of the 200 considered hair color one of the things that make them think someone is old. Wrinkles were checked only slightly more frequently. However, the way people moved turned out to be a significant measurement. Almost every one of those surveyed considered becoming inactive, stooped, unsteady, having poor posture, and walking slowly the most common characteristics of "old." So, now you know. Youthful, erect, confident, sprightly movement is a hallmark of those who put old on hold. I hope these positive words describe you.

Have you ever reclined on a slant board? If you haven't, you don't know what you are missing. You can make one inexpensively. Go to the lumberyard and ask them to cut a piece of plywood heavy enough to support your weight, long enough to lie on and wide enough for your body. Securely prop up one end about 12 inches from the floor. Put a mat or rug on it and stretch out on it (feet on the elevated end) for 30 minutes. The results are amazing. You defy gravity and everything goes back into place, including your facial muscles. Let yourself fall into a state of total relaxation and calm. It can be an effective non-medicinal tranquilizer. You can also use the slant board to do exercises to help strengthen and flatten your stomach muscles. (Strong abdominals will help ward off back problems.) A slant board is a versatile and dynamite put old on hold Super Key. You get so much benefit for little effort. Check with your doctor if you think using a slant board may not be right for you.

13 "Putting off Aging" by Betty Weir Alderson, *Rx Remedy*, May/June 2000

A slant board has been very helpful for my husband. His feet hurt most of the time and doctors can't figure out what's causing the problem. The usual culprits, such as arthritis and diabetes, have been ruled out. X-rays show nothing. Pain medication doesn't help. What does help is the slant board. When he rests on it, it's the only time he experiences pain relief. It's not uncommon for him to fall asleep on the board for a couple of hours and wake up refreshed.

Then there is yoga. In my thirties, as I mentioned earlier, I started doing yoga exercises with Richard Hittleman on TV. To this day the most comfortable way for me to sit is in the lotus position. It's an interesting thing about yoga: Even if you stop doing the positions on a regular basis, the body remembers what it learned long ago so it's easy to restart or continue stretching routines learned years earlier. Stretching should be a part of any exercise routine. With the popularity of yoga these days, classes, video tapes and DVDs are easy to find. Check with your doctor before starting a yoga exercise routine.

Facial exercise: Exercising the muscles in your face is just as important as exercising the rest of your body. There are many facial exercise books and regimens available but the one I like is Carol Maggio's Facercise program which you'll find listed in the Resources section. Maggio has a video in which she goes through a series of exercises with you.

Exercise your mind: One of the best mind and brain builders is crossword puzzles. Do them at every opportunity. Do them while you are watching mindless, boring TV, waiting for an appointment or enjoying a few minutes of down time. If you've never done one, don't start out with a difficult puzzle from the *New York Times*. Start with something easy and work your way up to the advanced level.

Read. Expand your knowledge base. Read books on a variety of topics. Choose reading materials that make you think or challenge you to expand your world view. Your brain is not nearly as overloaded as you might imagine. It holds a lot of room for you to grow into an even more interesting, knowledgeable, productive human being. A sharp, agile mind is a hallmark of one who has put old on hold.

Observe Others

Observation is a powerful teacher. Watch what people do that you consider aging behaviors or attitudes. For example, notice how people at different stages and ages dress and take care of personal grooming. Listen to how they speak and what they talk about. Watch how they move. Observing others will motivate you to monitor your own thinking, attitudes, and behaviors, and help do what's necessary to put old on hold. Be aware of the role of friends and family in shaping your thinking and behavior. People tend to mimic valued thinking and behaviors of those they associate with most often, so think about and monitor outside influences carefully. Be willing to venture beyond conventional thinking. Your example could encourage friends and family to embrace new ideas and practices, too.

Constantly Look for Inspiring Role Models

Your thinking and way of behaving develop in proportion to the number of positive stimulating images you see, so actively look for them. Constantly feeding your brain and subconscious with inspiring thoughts and pictures will positively influence your ability to put old on hold. In addition to wonderful role models in your own life, there are many veteran icons in the media to emulate.

Ageless TV personality Barbara Walters is inspiring. Like the Energizer Bunny, she keeps on going and gets better over time.

Then there is the amazing Carol Channing. Over age 80, and recently remarried, she's a perfect role model to inspire much older individuals who would like to fall in love again, but believing traditional wisdom, don't believe it's possible or perhaps even think it's inappropriate for those of advanced years. It appears she has discovered that love and happiness are better when you finally know what's important!

I am especially in awe of 84-year-old broadcaster Mike Wallace. I recently watched Mike being interviewed by journalist Tim Russert, and could not keep my eyes off the TV screen as I tried to figure out what makes Mike appear twenty years younger. Physically and mentally, he is unlike any 83-year-old I have ever seen. In most people his age such youthful animation, energy and sparkle no longer exist; instead, there are just dying dimly glowing coals, a fading image of what used to be.

In spite of a publicized bout with depression, he keeps on as if it never happened. Why the disparity between his chronological age and his physical appearance and outstanding mental agility? One reason may be that he is living seamlessly, continuing to grow because of his ongoing interaction with a variety of people. To my knowledge, he has never retired, even temporarily. Had he done so, I suspect he would have lost many of his youthful characteristics during that period.

Another explanation for his staying power may be his ability to look at events through what he calls fresh eyes. On another occasion I heard him mention how much he values the perspective of young people. This confirms my belief that to remain ageless, it's essential to maintain contact with younger people and appreciate what they offer. The point of view found in their fresh eyes could give balance and a new outlook to unintended inflexible thinking. It's not necessary to accept what those fresh eyes see or advocate. What's important is to be willing to try to understand how, what, and why those fresh eyes see as they do. This approach will help anyone stay as youthful as Mike Wallace.

How about Jack LaLanne. Thanks to Jack's exercise program on TV many years ago, I started working out in my thirties, along with the yoga. Accompanied by his beautiful white dog Happy, Jack was a mass of rippling muscles, oozing testosterone, bending and stretching, energetically jumping up and down, whistling and having a great time. I'll never forget his body-hugging jumpsuit that showed off his exquisitely chiseled physique and, above all, his pencil-slim hips. Oh, how I envied those hips!

I still do many of the hip-slimming exercises he did on his TV program. Has the effort been successful? If you ask my devoted husband, he will tell you I have the body of a goddess, but then, he's into science fiction. If you ask my friend Peggy, she will tell you my hips are to die for. But, given the circumference of her hips, she's ready to die for any hips that are even a tad tighter than hers are. The truth is, I do not have Jack's pencil-slim hips, but that's okay because I'm a work in progress. I will never stop trying, thanks to the enduring inspiration of this great role model.

Jack achieved his good health and physical condition through consistent hard work and unrelenting determination. I doubt he relied on the kind of gimmicky paraphernalia sold by exercise gurus today. On his program, Jack used a chair to help perform exercises. He didn't sell pricey exercise gadgets that quickly end up in a garage sale. To help with stretching, he did sell an inexpensive rubber cord that looked like a jump rope, which I bought, still have, and consider as good as new (like Jack himself).

If you've seen him on TV recently, you know what a phenomenon he is. Now in his eighties, he's just as tight and trim as ever and, yes, he still has those pencil-slim hips and still oozes testosterone. He's a powerful inspiration. When I see him I think, "Gee, when I get to be his age, I can look and feel just as good as he does." You have no idea how great it feels at age seventy-plus to be able to say, "When I get to be his age . . ." To have something wonderful to look forward to achieving can be a great motivator. Jack proves that a second life exists for those who want it and are willing to do what it takes to get it. I hope he lives forever!

Have you seen and heard singer Tony Bennett lately? Now over 70, he's still going strong. His voice is every bit as powerful as in his younger days and his appearance belies his chronological age. Catch the sparkle in his eyes that confirms he's still got it going on. Every guy should wear as well as he has.

Start keeping a journal or scrapbook of people who inspire you, documenting which characteristics motivate you to reach your goals. Review your list frequently and continue to add ageless heroes to it. The more role models you have, the better. Staying aware of the success of others will help you achieve your goals. If they can do it, you can too.

Be a Positive Role Model Yourself

Help others grow to be ageless. Discover the "youthifying" power in the feedback you receive when you make a difference in someone else's life. Giving of yourself is the ultimate selfishness because you, the giver, always receive more than the recipient does.

Here's an example of a super youthifying experience. The September, 2000 issue of *Life Extension* magazine published an article about me. In a letter to the editor the following month, a woman wrote to say how much she appreciated learning about me and how much it helped her. When I first read that wonderful letter, my endorphins kicked into high gear because I realized how positively I had touched the life of another. I felt wonderful. I am convinced that, for a brief period of time after I read her letter, any aging had stopped and regeneration had taken place in my body. I encourage you to have as many positive, giving, youthifying experiences as possible. It's the closest thing to real magic you will ever know. And I personally invite you to let me know how this book helps you put old on hold; that way we will both benefit.

Maintain an Inventory of Your Skills

Constantly evaluate your mental and physical abilities. Keep a running inventory of skills you consider important for staying young. Take steps to maintain and improve them. For example, can you still:

- Breathlessly climb a flight of stairs?
- Walk as quickly as you did a year ago?
- Bend and touch your toes?

Was there anything you could do even six months ago you can no longer do? If so, can you regain that ability with some effort?

If a skill or ability has diminished or is seemingly lost, please don't assume it's gone forever. If you lost a particular youthful characteristic by default (meaning through laziness or inattention), start working slowly to get it back. Be defiant about it. Don't tell yourself "it's too late" or "I'm too far gone." Just work at it consistently and persistently! I cannot begin to tell you how little victories will build your self-esteem. They add up, quicker than you can imagine and you will come to a place in your life and in your mind where you will see yourself in an entirely different light. So will others. People will comment positively on the evolving you.

I challenge you to take a systematic approach to get to where you want to be. Make a plan then take action. Do something to move toward your goal every day. It works, and each step of improvement, positively reinforced by others as your progress becomes visible, propels you toward your goal. You will thrive on the positive feedback you'll receive. It's a self-perpetuating process.

Defy Convention: Be a Rebel with a Cause

In your journal or scrapbook, make a list of age-related taboos, the activities, ideas, or behaviors that others might criticize or disparage. For example, would you like to take acting or voice lessons because, even at your supposed advanced age, you still yearn to be a professional entertainer? In some families and communities, an older, seemingly settled person is considered on the brink of senility for even entertaining such a dream, let alone trying to make it a reality. In my own family, I can recall when my oldest sister, in her thirties, told my mother she wanted to learn how to tap dance. Mom's negative response devastated my sister. The subject never came up again and, of course, my sister never learned to tap dance for fear of incurring Mom's disapproval.

Would you like to run for public office but fear public opinion might shoot you down because of your age? Ronald Reagan and Robert Dole were among the first to suffer the arrows of ageism, but they persisted. You can, too. Would you like to be a flight attendant, a job traditionally held by young people? This profession is wide open today. It's no longer necessary to be an attractive blonde female under the age of 25. Your friends and family may think you are crazy, but so what?

Would you like to have a relationship with an older/younger person or with someone from another race or culture, but put it out of your mind because of how it would look at your age? Ask yourself if behaviors, ideas, or activities you are considering would qualify as illegal, immoral, or unethical. Would they harm others or burden your conscience? If not, go for it. Challenge the fear. Step up to the plate and take a swing at irrational cultural, traditional, or social no-nos. Even if you are booed by onlookers (who may secretly admire your daring), so what? It is both exhilarating and liberating to overcome obstacles. Dare to challenge the status quo. Defying convention is an effective tool to put old on hold.

Believe me when I say you are not too old to do what you want. If not now, when? Napoleon Hill said what your mind can conceive, you can achieve. The truth in that adage, heard so often, may have lost its originality, but I want you to adopt it as a mantra. Silently repeat these words any time you are afraid to try something new because of your age. You know within what you are capable of doing. "I'm too old to do that" should never cross your mind, let alone your lips.

Remember, growing old is a choice. The alternative is staying ageless. You can suspend the aging process if you have a plan and do what it takes to stay in control of your health, thoughts, behavior, and speech. As early in life as possible, choose to think and do what will enhance your health and longevity. Use this book as a guide and you'll make it. I could use your company.

Cultivate a Sense of Humor and a Realistic Perspective

The stuff you fret and fume about today won't even be a blur in your mind next week, so don't sweat it. So what if the dry cleaner loses your favorite shirt. It happened to me, and I wasted a whole week being angry. But guess what: Now I don't even remember what the shirt looked like. The world is full of terrific shirts, so I bought a new one. Was the lost garment worth fuming and fussing over? No, because there was nothing I could do to get it back. Sue the dry cleaner, maybe. I'm kidding, of course. At times like this, a sense of humor and a reality check come in handy.

Prepare yourself to accept the realities of life. Unfortunate things do indeed happen to nice people and that's the way life is. The shirt I fumed over was small stuff. Looking at life in retrospect and realizing how silly we behave in a given situation should, ideally, happen only rarely. Learn to spot the small stuff situations when they happen, deal with them immediately in a calm, rational manner, and then get on with more positive things in your life. Don't allow yourself to behave like a self-absorbed jerk. When a small stuff situation happens, and, as Richard Carlson says, it's all small stuff, question if it will likely be a major issue next week. Be brutally honest and ask yourself if you'll even remember it happened. People who put old on hold keep things in perspective and live by this principle. It defuses a lot of stress and avoids unnecessary grief. The bonus: You'll have fewer worry lines engraved on your face and more happy sparkles in your eyes.

Be Kind and Patient

It's simply the Golden Rule: Be kind and tolerant, particularly with those you love and especially with those from whom you want or need something. It seems odd that elderly people, retirees in particular, don't like to wait. They don't have a bus or plane to catch; they don't have to be some place at a specific time, but if made to wait, they can get very cranky. I used to say it's because the portion of the brain that controls civilized behavior has turned to concrete, but it's more complex than that.

More likely, cantankerous behavior could result from physical pain or discomfort, or hardening of the arteries that impairs blood flow to the brain. Or it may just be a lifelong character defect that surfaces when people no longer care what others think. It may also result from bitterness and remorse over an unfulfilled life. It may be a manifestation of depression. Too much or unnecessary medication or even alcoholism may play a role. More than a few seniors have told me they drink to dull their painful arthritis or to blank out an unhappy, lonely existence.

For men, I think hormone decline negatively exacerbates personality changes, at least in part. Earlier I spoke about getting an annual comprehensive blood test called the CBC/Chemistry profile. This is not just for women; men need it, too. It can uncover potential problems, including hormonal, that once corrected can result in a dramatic, positive personality change. But diminished testosterone doesn't affect all men equally. Some stay rational, but others become belligerent.

My way of dealing with difficult people is to get to know them on a first-name basis. Some of the crankiest people become completely rational when you establish a one-to-one relationship with them. It has proven to me that it's not old age or hardened arteries or hormone loss that cause objectionable behavior, it's choice. People decide how they want to behave. It's as simple as that. And old people seem to make more negative behavior choices than young people. Maybe they're just not paying attention.

Resolve right now that you will always be a class act in the deportment department. It will go a long way toward helping you put old on hold. Stay aware of how your behavior may be changing and make a conscious effort to be rational at all times. If you have all your mental faculties intact, you can control your behavior. It will have a tremendously positive effect on the way others see and treat you.

Wear a Pleasant Expression

Discover the youthifying power that comes with a pleasant expression. It's not just the artistic quality of the Mona Lisa that captivates. It's the smile! Keep the corners of your mouth upturned in a Mona Lisa smile and it will keep you looking young. When you smile, you are more attractive, there is a sparkle in your eyes, and it's easier to think pleasant thoughts. Smiling also lowers blood pressure, boosts metabolism and endorphin levels, and reduces tension. Yeah!

When out in the mall, try this experiment. As you pass people, make eye contact with your Mona Lisa smile in place and watch them smile back, sometimes with big toothy smiles. You'll make their day and their response will make yours. Try this with babies. In their innocence, they recognize beauty in a friendly face and react accordingly. What is more wonderful than the beaming face of a baby in response to your warm smiling countenance? It's positive proof that a smile works wonders. When you have a pleasant look on your face you are open, inviting and non-threatening. It's a no-sweat way to help you and others put old on hold. A possible bonus: You may even meet someone wonderful.

Don't Play Age Games

If you think you look great for your age, please don't invite others to guess how old you are. It's a dead giveaway you're an old fogey desperate for a compliment. No one needs to know how old you are. Don't ask "how old do you think I am" as a reality check to see how you are doing or how others perceive you. Use your mirror instead, or observe how others respond to you, particularly young people. By simple observation, you can see for yourself how you are perfecting the art of agelessness. Remember, the point is not to be dwelling on age numbers, anyway.

Alternatively, don't volunteer your age. I had a customer who really looked great for his age, but he became a nuisance because every time we saw him, he boasted about how old he was. He may have looked good, but his behavior told everyone he was an old goat, begging for accolades.

Say You Feel Terrific

If you have health problems, keep them between you and your doctor. When you feel needy or burdened make an appointment and unload everything on a professional. This may come as a shock, but most people (not even friends) are not interested in the details of your angioplasty or how you nearly died in the operating room. They will listen politely and make all the appropriate empathy noises, but they would rather hear something else. When someone asks, "How are you?" please understand it's not an open invitation to share your woes. Make your answer a superlative such as "I'm terrific!" It will make others happier to see you. You'll feel better and so will they. This is a good place for me to remind you that your subconscious accepts everything you say about yourself as gospel. Imagine the effects of a whole day of "Oh, I'm not feeling well" or "I'm feeling great!"

Keep Your Appearance Contemporary

If public slovenliness and partial nudity bothers you as much as it does me, please join my crusade to reestablish even semi good taste in dressing. (This offer is for men as well as women!) What's good taste? Nobody seems to know anymore, but I think most of us over the age of twenty have a wee small voice within that whispers, "That looks awful," or "You shouldn't be seen in public looking like that." If you hear that voice within or if someone who loves you cares enough to tell you the truth, pay attention. Adapt, don't automatically adopt what's current if it's not your style or is clearly inappropriate. (My crystal ball tells me that the next accepted fashion will be to go topless. Bodies are already bare at beaches and in bars – what's the logical progression?) Wear what's appropriate and pegs you as a model of an ageless god or goddess.

One day I was both amused and horrified to see an overweight Boomer, long salt-and-pepper hair (mostly yellowish white) in a ponytail, wearing a revealing low-cut, cut-off tank top. The rolls of fat hanging over her too-tight jeans were something to behold. I marveled at how she could think she looked sexy or in style; why else would she venture out of the house looking like that? The whole image was a calling card that screamed, "I'm an aging Boomer in denial. Even if I look ridiculous, this is my way of staying young." Wear what you believe is right for you, but remember, the key is to look ageless. This means that every aspect of the picture is tasteful and complementary, with no aspect drawing overt attention.

Skinny teenagers may look cute with an exposed belly button, pierced or not, but I don't look cute with my belly button hanging out and neither does any mature woman, even if she's looking like Demi Moore. Flab-free teens may look cute in their short shorts. I don't, so I spare others the visual insult by covering up. Besides, I believe in mystery. I would much rather have others wonder what it looks like "under there." (For the record, my devoted husband would say it's phenomenal. You'll just have to take his word for it!)

Be a head turner in the best sense of the word. Reward others who are head turners. When you see others who look great, tell them. You'll be sure to make their day and yours as well. One day while in line at a supermarket, I noticed a woman in another checkout line who looked terrific, as if she had spent time thinking about her appearance. She wasn't overdone; she just looked well put together. I asked the person behind me to hold my place, and then I went over to her and said, "I just wanted to tell you that you look wonderful." She lit up like a thousand-watt light bulb. Her husband standing beside her beamed with pride, and nearly popped his shirt buttons. She thanked me profusely for making her day. Her reaction made my day as well. Sure, it's risky to walk up to people and comment on their appearance; they can always tell you to go away and mind your own business, but who in their right mind would? Most people welcome kind comments from a stranger if they're sincere, respectful and not intrusive.

Make it a practice to constantly "upgrade" your appearance with little tweaks and enhancements here and there. It's like a computer. Your original version works fine but newer enhancements appear on the market like clockwork. Your computer may not need all the latest bells and whistles, but you'll want some of them. It's the same with you. While you don't want to latch on to every fashion fad that comes along, use the best of what's new to continually reinvent yourself with a look that continues to get better. I emphasize the importance of adapting rather than adopting. For example, if the latest thing in shoes makes your feet look deformed or pinches your toes, search for the best among the worst of the styles or wait until designers start liking women again, and they will, eventually.

If you don't constantly reinvent your appearance, you will forever look as if you are stuck in the sixties, seventies, or whatever. Don't wait for your kids or spouse to suggest you need a makeover. Use what is available in the fashion world that will transform you into a head turner. Remember, when you look contemporary, you look ageless – another great tool to help you put old on hold. Will you be inviting envy? Maybe, but you'll also be doing a good deed. You will be inspiring your friends and peers to be their best. That's a win-win situation!

Consider Medical and Dental Enhancement

Whether you choose to have cosmetic surgery of any kind, be it a facelift, breast augmentation, or liposuction depends on how satisfied you are with your appearance. It's an extremely personal decision, as well as a costly one. You should not allow anyone to talk you in or out of it. If you opt for cosmetic surgery, do so only after thorough research. To help you do it right, you'll find Susan Gail's book, *Cosmetic Surgery: Before, Between and After* in the Resources section. It's a necessary read before you make a decision.

What you see in the mirror, how you perceive yourself, how you think you appear to the world affects your thinking and behavior. It will have a bearing on how well you ultimately put old on hold. I suggest you go about any cosmetic improvement in a thoughtful, organized way. For example, when I was just a kid of 69, I decided to get braces on my teeth. It was a wonderful experience. Let me explain how it came about.

I was born with teeth like Cher's, if you recall what hers looked like before she had them fixed. I grew up hating my teeth, believing no one could possibly love me because they were so unattractive. Fortunately, my husband looked beyond my imperfect smile and recognized the budding goddess there. When dental bonding first became available, I was ecstatic. I could finally do something about those ugly teeth. (Bonding is the application of plastic material to existing teeth to fill in spaces, make teeth wider or longer, or make other corrections.) Bonding helped a good deal, but it wasn't the ultimate answer because in time bonding wears off and you are right back where you started.

The last dentist I consulted suggested braces as a first step to improvement. I thought he was crazy. And let me point out that my thinking that he was crazy is a perfect example of how tradition, custom, and expectation influence thinking. After all, was there another human being on earth with teeth in braces at age sixty-nine? At the urging of my loving, supportive husband who would deny this goddess nothing, I decided to go for it. Later on, I learned I was not a trendsetter. Others much older than I had braces on their teeth. I read about a woman, 90, in a nursing home who had her teeth straightened. A waste of time and money you might think? Who cares? It's her life, her teeth, her budget and, frankly, I think it's great. Who knows how long she will live? Regardless, it will enhance her quality of life and make her more attractive and feel better about herself. Even 90-year-olds, or especially them, deserve a boost in self esteem. Such a high percentage of old people have unattractive teeth; you don't want them to kiss you, even on your cheek.

Without question, opting for braces was the absolute first best thing I could have done to improve my appearance. It took 18 months of discomfort and tolerating the unsightly train tracks that others had to look at. But it was well worth the trouble. Seeing all that bothersome metal in my mouth at my advanced age positively inspired mothers of teenagers in braces to go for them for themselves. After all, if I wasn't too old, neither were they! This is another example of how delightful it feels to be a positive influence on others.

I recall only one disheartening experience. One of my friends, older than I, inspired by my braces, asked her dentist (not an orthodontist) if he thought she'd be a candidate for braces. Nasty man that he was, he told her it would be "impractical at your age." She was so devastated that she just accepted his uninformed opinion. Don't ever allow anyone to shoot down your dreams and aspirations. Go for a second opinion. You can most always find an ethical, skilled, open-minded professional to provide what you are looking for. Remember, defying convention is second nature to those who put old on hold! Braces for older people may invite disapproving glances, but who cares? Braces are neither illegal nor immoral, so if you want your teeth in heavy metal, go for it! And just for the record, heavy metal is not all there is. Now there is everything from clear non-braces to more esthetically pleasing appliances that are hardly apparent.

I always intended to have some cosmetic surgery, but getting my teeth straightened was a priority. It seemed a waste of money to get a facelift without first fixing my teeth. In going through "before" and "after" photos in cosmetic surgeons' offices, I wondered why surgeons don't work with orthodontists. They'd be doing their cosmetic surgery patients a huge favor if they encouraged them to take care of their teeth first, or even after surgery, for that matter. Better late than never.

Having jumped the braces hurdle, it was time to move on to the next phase, so I had cosmetic surgery, a face lift. Not that I needed it, you understand. I remind you that if you want to put old on hold, it requires preventive maintenance, interior and exterior. Think of your body as the home you live in; that's where you will dwell for as long as you live. You can't move and find a better one; you have to constantly take care of what you have. When the stucco (your skin) starts to crack and peel you have it repaired. When the roof of your home (your face) starts to sag you don't wait for it to cave in before you fix it! So I fix needed repairs as I go along. Am I glad I had surgery? Absolutely. My husband says you should see me now. He's not unhappy that I look twenty years younger than he does, since I am two years older!

Attractiveness, however you define it, begins on the inside. Surgery can only do so much; you can limit the amount of surgery needed by controlling what you ingest and what you think about, believe, and act upon, over a long period of time. It's unfortunate to see people spend money on all kinds of creams, potions and cosmetic applications trying to put off or hide the ravages of time yet they continue to eat palate-pleasing junk that destroys youth and accelerates aging.

The physical aspect of putting old on hold is pretty simple. Assuming you are not afflicted with a birth defect, or difficult to control medical condition, if you take care of your health, maintain a positive, determined attitude, and drink adequate amounts of water, then your appearance will be better than average far longer than you can imagine.

Watch Your Posture

Pay attention to your posture. If you are exercising, watching your diet, building your strength and having yearly tests for osteoporosis, you should be standing tall. Visualize the hands of a clock at the stroke of 6:00. That's the posture you want: Knees over the ankles, your hips over your knees, your shoulders over your hips and your head erect, between your shoulders. You know you are losing it when you see yourself moving to 6:10, 6:15 and so on. Keep your shoulders slightly back. Sit tall, stand tall, walk tall, think tall. When you see someone with poor posture, use it as a cue to readjust your posture. Think goddess or princess. Visualize carrying yourself with the regal bearing of Princess Grace of Monaco or Audrey Hepburn as she so elegantly carried herself in the movie *Roman Holiday*. Those are my posture role models, visualize who works for you. For men, remember Yul Brynner and Sean Connery? Two upright guys! The world will look more inviting as you stand tall, and you will look better, too! Remember, good posture is a highly youthful characteristic.

Visualize Your Future

Develop and continually refine your plan to grow ageless. Visualize how you want to be and look 10 years from now. Make the plan clear and vivid, with great detail. Write down what you will do and how you will put your plan into action. If you doubt the value of visualization, let me tell you about a new study conducted by a team of Yale researchers[14]. This research excites me because it confirms everything I've ever believed, thought about, or practiced in my life.

---

14 "Longevity Increased by Positive Self-Perceptions of Aging," Becca R. Levy, et al, Yale University. Published in *Journal of Personality and Social Psychology*, 2002, Vol 83, No. 2, 261–270

Among other things, the researchers found that individuals acquire age stereotypes several decades before becoming old. Thus, younger individuals are likely to automatically accept age stereotypes without questioning their validity. That means if you want to put old on hold, you have to know what you want to look like when you are "old" and never lose sight of your vision. I have never lost sight of my vision, but then, I had great but unintended motivation. Here's how it came about:

I am child number five in a family of seven. By the time I came along, my mother had gray hair and looked grandmotherly. (In other words, she looked old.) None of the mothers of my friends looked old. Only mine. To make matters worse, she always, and I do mean always, complained about not feeling well. As a result, I constantly worried she would die before I grew up and that bothered me a lot. It was on my mind constantly. We did not have an extended family and there were no close family friends or even casual ones who would have made an acceptable mother substitute. My mother's premature aging and poor health bothered me so profoundly that I vowed I would never get old. At 10 years of age this wasn't a passing childhood fancy. I was obsessed. I didn't have a clue how I would do it, but I knew what I wanted to look like when I got to my mother's age. I saw a picture in a magazine of a pretty young mother with her two young children. This was my image. I *knew* this was how I wanted to look.

To this day, the picture of that young woman is as sharp in my mind as it was 65 years ago. I am convinced that who I am and how I look and feel today is the result of holding on to that mental picture, I always saw myself as that young woman. If asked how old I am inside there is no question, I am thirty. I don't feel old. I've never felt old. When I hear a woman, perhaps 10 years younger than I complain, "I feel so old," I simply can't relate to that feeling. Now you can fully understand why I am so excited about the Yale study. It validates my belief that what you envision through out your life has power beyond what you might imagine. Because of always holding that young vision in mind, I think I intuitively made choices very early on that supported and moved me toward my goal of agelessness.

Because of conclusions drawn in the Yale study, I've given a good deal of thought to the consciousness of inner age. My husband, who is chronologically two years younger than I am, says that inside he feels fifty-five. Why does he feel 55 while I feel thirty? What was going on in my life when I was 30 that never allowed me to age beyond that number as my perceived inner age? I still hold in memory that picture of that thirty-ish young woman from my childhood. What role did this image play in my feeling "forever thirty?" Just about anyone you ask who is in good health will tell you that deep inside they feel a specific number of years younger than they are chronologically. Why is this so? Could it be that perceived inner age corresponds to a clearly defined mental picture or a physical state of being that existed at a specific age? Does that become your inner age in later years, shaping your thinking and behavior? I believe it does. I believe that awareness of inner age is extremely powerful and increasingly important over time. It gives permission and encouragement to think, behave, and function as one might at that chronological age.

For whatever reason, it represents a strong explicit manifestation of how young or old you really are.

Do you have a mental picture of how you want to look or how you will be when you are 60, 70, and beyond? Do you envision yourself as slim and agile, healthy and strong, with an erect posture? What will your hair, face, and teeth look like? How will you be dressed? What will you be doing that is challenging and productive? What activities and work will engage your mind and time? What kind of people will you be living, working or associating with, and in what circumstances? What goals will you be accomplishing? Will you have what matters most to you? I hope you will spend some time reflecting on and answering these questions. Doing so can have a profound effect on your future state of being.

Constantly refine your future image and circumstances until they become so real you will grow into them as a matter of course. Let your subconscious automatically steer you toward what you visualize for yourself. You will become what you think about most persistently and consistently, not because I say so, but because that's ultimately how your brain works. We gravitate toward our dominant thoughts. Accepting this reality will lead you to make many positive changes in your life. It's impossible for me to emphasize how important it is for you to grasp that the quality and quantity of your thoughts are extremely powerful. Most people miss the significance. I sincerely hope you get it.

Now is the perfect time to take stock of what goes on in your head. Be brutally honest with yourself and, at the same time, be kind. Don't beat yourself up if you come to the realization that you are plagued with negative thoughts. Acknowledge what you do and don't like about your thinking habits, resolve to change what you don't like, then do it. The process is slow, but that doesn't matter. Over time, you're the winner. Keep working to establish your ideal inner age, and I guarantee that eventually you will succeed. Here's a suggestion: Every time you catch yourself thinking a negative thought, replace it with a positive one. Soon you'll be correcting yourself automatically.

Begin now and be persistent. Prioritize. Develop an anti-aging program and happily do it each day, even and especially, when you don't feel like it. This is the key to success: Relentless persistence, regardless of what is going on in your head or your life. I know from experience it works. If I can do it you can do it. Start today.

Just Say No to the Deadly Sins of Negative Self Talk

There is no way to put this gently, so I won't try: Negative self-talk is destructive. If you fully realized how it hastens decline, you wouldn't indulge in it. When I hear someone's negative statements, I automatically assume the persona of Judge Judy at her meanest. I become preachy and pious. At that point, I am not above chastising a perfect stranger (with a bit of a smile, of course) for assaulting my ears with the utterance of sinful negative self talk.

Excuse me for a moment as I climb to my pulpit so I can do some preaching. I want to hear your "Amen!" loud and clear in agreement as I deliver my sermon.

"Brothers and sisters, we are gathered here together to learn how to put old on hold. If you want salvation from debilitating old age, if you desire the blissful state of agelessness, you will avoid committing the Seven Deadly Sins of Negative Self Talk. Confess the sins you have committed, do the penance prescribed, and move on to enjoy the blessings of a long, healthy productive life."

Here are the Seven Deadly Sins of Negative Self Talk:

- I must be getting old.
- I'm having a "senior moment."
- I'm too old to (learn) (do) that.
- I'm just an old broad (old geezer).
- I'm a senior and deserve special treatment.
- My brain (body) isn't what it used to be.
- I don't have the time, energy, imagination to put old on hold. I'm too tired to even think about it.

Let's look at each of these transgressions and how they can cast you into an unnecessary state of "old age hell":

DEADLY SIN # 1: "I must be getting old"

How often have you said or thought, "I must be getting old" when you do something klutzy or feel a kink in your back? The effect is devastating – not that you dropped something or feel a catch in your body, but that you chastise yourself for being like everybody else, regardless of age. Negative self-talk will transport you down the road to decline, deterioration, and decrepitude faster than you can imagine. If you want to put old on hold, don't beat up on yourself for exhibiting human frailty or having an occasional body twinge.

Your subconscious mind is so powerful and obedient. It listens to and internalizes everything you say or think about. Your subconscious also takes to heart negative comments others make about you. It believes what it hears unless you immediately reject or correct what it hears. Visualize your subconscious as an officious, haughty English butler who doesn't judge thoughts or intentions, but whose duty is to fulfill every perceived directive or desire, and he executes his duty with precision and perfection. Be careful what your brain butler hears you or others say about you, so that what goes on in your head is as nourishing and healthy as what you put into your body.

For your penance: Next time you drop something or feel a little twinge, don't tell yourself you are getting old. Get a new attitude! Bend over, pick it up, and focus on how good it feels to be able to bend and stretch. If it feels especially good, drop the item again and pick it up with the other hand so you get a better workout.

DEADLY SIN # 2: "I'm having a senior moment"

Misplace or forget something? Draw a blank with someone's name or a movie title? Be patient with yourself instead of immediately chastising yourself about getting old or having a "senior moment." Don't assume you have Alzheimer's or that you are losing it until and unless an expert diagnoses the condition. Don't get frustrated and try to force yourself to remember. Relax. Your brain is having a traffic jam. It will clear and come to you eventually.

If something has eluded you all day, right before you go to bed, think about it; even write it down, and ask your subconscious to help you remember. The answer may come to you in the middle of the night when you get up and go to the bathroom. Your mind will be relaxed, allowing the answer to pop into your head. This isn't magic, new age or esoteric. Your mind and body will do your bidding if you give it a chance. In between these occasions, don't tell yourself you are getting old. Instead, say you're getting better. By relaxing and allowing, instead of resisting these moments, you'll experience fewer such lapses and you will enhance your ability to put old on hold at the same time.

For your penance: I'm going to go easy on you with this one. It's traumatic enough to unnecessarily think you are losing your mind. The next time you have a memory lapse, just remember that young people forget things all the time and they don't blame a momentary mental snafu on having a "junior moment." Relax and give your brain a chance to regroup and give you the information you want.

DEADLY SIN # 3: "I'm too old to (learn) (do) that"

Condemning yourself as too old to do or learn offends your abilities and places limits on your potential. I'll wager that you engage in this sin not because you really believe you are too old, but because you think it's what you are supposed to say at your age. You have a strong sense of what you are capable of doing, so chronological age be damned. You're not going to get any younger so you may as well go for it now.

Here's an example to illustrate my point. The wife of a coworker and friend died suddenly. While working together, he would talk about all the Walter Mitty things he wanted to do, such as sailing, hang gliding, and other daring activities. He never attempted those activities because his wife discouraged him. Her reaction was understandable; she was concerned for his safety. Some time after her death, he wrote me a note telling me what he was up to. His list of activities included more than a few of the forbidden fruit things he had always wanted to do. Then, in parentheses, he added the words, "I guess I should be acting my age." At age 52? I don't think so! Being his friend, I verbally smacked him on the side of the head a couple of times, and I suspect he will never again think he is too old to do whatever he wants to do and knows he *can* do.

I often hear an older person say they are too old to learn when faced with a new challenge. When a new computer program was installed at work, a pharmacist some few years my junior complained, "I'm too old to be learning this." No, he's not too old. Lazy, perhaps, but not too old. Age has nothing to do with our ability to learn.

For your penance: If you consider yourself too old to learn, sign up for a class to learn something you believe you are "too old" to learn. Your success will make you feel younger, bolster your self-esteem, and increase your faith in your ability to tackle anything you put your mind to, regardless of your age.

Get a notebook and write out two positive affirmations for every negative "I can't or shouldn't . . ." that comes into your head. Forget whatever traditions, expectations, customs, or the opinion of family or well-meaning friends who are only too quick to caution about what you shouldn't do at your age. Think of why you *should* do it and write a firm, positive statement to that effect. Read this statement as many times as it takes to give permission or help you to find the courage to do what you want. It's entirely your call.

DEADLY SIN # 4: "I'm just an old broad (old geezer)"

Please, if you want to stay on my good side, don't ever refer to yourself as an old broad or old geezer. If you do, I'll hunt you down, call Judge Judy, and have you committed to a retirement community where you can miserably commiserate with real old broads and geezers and others like them.

These terms are dreadfully demeaning. In 2001, a TV film titled *These Old Broads* starred Elizabeth Taylor, 68, Shirley MacLaine, 66, and Debbie Reynolds, 68, in which they mocked themselves and their public images. It was sad. These women are not old broads but worse, their portrayal as such gave the term legitimacy.

For your penance: Don't wait for the next time the conditioned reflex to call yourself an old broad kicks in. Look in a mirror several times a day and acknowledge the vitality and dynamic spirit you exude. What you see is not an old broad or geezer, and don't you forget it.

Girlfriend, every morning, put on your best face, get dressed and prepare to astound the world with your ageless uniqueness. Pretend that the debonair movie star Fernando Lamas, the legendary charming rascal, is next to you, cooing into you ear the same outrageous line he handed every woman he met, "Dahling, you look mah-vel-ous." If you have never heard of Fernando Lamas, it doesn't matter. His appreciation of feminine pulchritude made women feel special and that is what counts. Don't ever leave the house without telling yourself how "mah-vel-ous" you are. Every woman has a goddess within and so do you. Don't ever forget it.

For the guys, I want you to do a similar mirror exercise. Every time you look in a mirror, stand tall, suck in your gut and tell yourself what a handsome devil (god) you are. I'll be there watching over your shoulder. I, the ultimate goddess of ageless goddesses, will be there to encourage you on your journey to healthy agelessness. Just be sure to keep your hair short, out of your nose and ears, trim the scraggly eyebrows and get rid of all hair on your face. (It's not cool to strain your soup through an overgrown mustache or have it drip into a bacteria-harboring beard, you know!) Nothing ages an older guy more than hair where it doesn't belong. If you don't sense that I'm there watching over you, it's probably because you've broken one of my commandments. But you can always repent, you understand, and I'll be back to cheer you on.

DEADLY SIN # 5: "I'm a senior and I deserve special consideration"

The age at which one becomes officially designated a "senior" is dropping to 55 and even younger, so it's not uncommon for Boomers to fall into the sin of entitlement early in the aging process. Our culture promotes the idea that with age comes privilege. Regardless of accepted norms, once you perceive yourself as deserving special consideration because of your age and for no other good reason, you have stooped to ageist sinfulness.

In this part of the sermon let me remind you it's only by the grace of God that you are living so long. Is this not reward enough? Why expect anything special simply for reaching 50, 60, 70, or beyond? Even if you've taken excellent care of your health, you still can't take full credit for your longevity. You've been lucky. Life can end in an instant, regardless of how you have lived.

Asking for or expecting special treatment invites sympathy, and, as you age that's the last thing you need or want. It encourages development of a scarcity mentality. You start to imagine your age entitles you to special consideration, so you begin to act accordingly. Pretty soon you expect special treatment and when you don't get it you get cranky or put out.

In addition, hard-up behavior affects how others regard and treat you. Once you start asking for something you don't really need or deserve, it undermines your self-respect and hastens the decline of your personal power. If you are already campaigning for special treatment wherever you go, stop before it becomes a deeply ingrained habit. Don't begin to see age-related rewards as a right or entitlement. Self-respect is more important than asking for or taking what you don't really need.

Here's a fair warning to you, my aging brothers and sisters: If I catch you at the fast food emporium groveling for senior coffee and your Mercedes, Lexus, or Jaguar is parked outside, your tires may be flat when you are ready to leave! I'd report you to Judge Judy but I don't think she has come up with a sentence harsh enough for this offense.

For your penance: Spend at least 10 minutes a day being grateful for the gift of longevity and use it to help others less fortunate than you. Stifle that sense of entitlement by going out of your way to help truly needy individuals get the assistance they need. Use your luxury car or old jalopy to transport needy persons to the fast food place where they can enjoy their senior coffee. And last, by example, encourage others to have an independent can-do attitude.

DEADLY SIN # 6: "My brain (body) isn't want it used to be"

No kidding! Whose body is what it used to be? We all change as we age. But we have the power to control how aging progresses. We can take supplements to enhance and maintain mental sharpness and we can exercise to stay in shape. Bottom line: Those who value what they were born with work at keeping it. It's not a big deal; you can do it!

For your penance: Take stock of your mental and physical condition as it is. Decide that you value what you have and you are not going to allow time and negligent habits to rob you of your life. Each day make one change in your diet that will help you lose weight or make you feel or function better. Begin to de-gunk your arteries and body by giving up fatty chips or any greasy ingestible that is aging you prematurely. Spend just two minutes a day doing simple bending and stretching. As it becomes a regular part of your life spend more time on it and move on to other forms of exercise, like walking.

DEADLY SIN # 7: "I don't have the time, energy, or imagination to put old on hold. I'm too tired to even think about it"

Okay, when you wake up from your self-induced coma, start to think about what your life will be like in your so-called golden years, assuming you live long enough to reach that point. You have time to do whatever you really want to do. If you are satisfied with your health and life the way it is, then that's a decision you have made. If, on the other hand, you would really like to have the energy and experience the joy of living agelessly, you will start to think about it and act on it. There is enough information in this book to get you started.

For your penance: There is none. You are living your penance right now if you are too tired, or too lazy to take charge of your life. But I'm not giving up on you. You are a valuable human being who deserves better. Please readjust your attitude about yourself in spite of what may be going on in your life that is dragging you down. Do one small thing each day that will bring to light the god or goddess you really are. I don't care what kind of shape you are in at this moment; you can overcome! You are better and more capable than you think.

Avoiding The Seven Deadly Sins of Negative Self Talk will help make your pilgrimage to agelessness so much smoother. The sins mentioned here aren't the only obstacles. Be aware of them, rebuke them, and avoid them as you would the plague. Lovingly chastise others who are guilty of committing them. Remind yourself and others that to achieve healthy agelessness, saying negative things about yourself or harboring limited perceptions of what you can or cannot do flies in the face of putting old on hold.

Do Not Worship in the Church of Chronological Age

We're not done with the sermon yet, brothers and sisters. Open up your hearts and minds as we cover the last of the transgressions. Before I move away from the pulpit I feel moved to spread the word. Closely tied to the Deadly Sins of Negative Self Talk is the abominable Church of Chronological Age, an ever growing congregation of those who believe they are over the hill.

Years ago while doing legal research, I came across a case known as Torcaso v. Watkins. It established that belief in God was not necessary to consider a belief system to be a religion.

In thinking about how our society deals with age and the aging process, it occurred to me we do indeed have a religion of chronological age, with its tenets demanding a rigid code of thinking and behaving. It's an insidious religion because most people are unaware of their belief system until outsiders point it out. Major tenets of the Religion of Chronological Age are as follows:

- *Thou shall retire at 65 (or sooner) and look forward to a life of leisure.* This belief is changing but still hangs on tenaciously. The website www.retired.com celebrates the so-called admired status of being retired. I looked at the website and, after quickly assessing the shallowness of its premise, what popped into my mind was an old

Peggy Lee song, "Is That All There Is?" Food, travel, hobbies, relationships, all nice in their own realm, but as a way of life? Eventually, it has to seem superficial. Living life as a pastime sucks the vitality from our veins and invites rapid decline.

- *Thou shall joke about thy age and refer to thyself as "old" at every opportunity. Thy friends will love thee for thy honesty because it makes them feel better about their own downward spiral.* One of the reasons self-deprecating remarks are accepted is because it offers a sense of kinship and comradeship. It confirms membership in this special congregation called the Church of Chronological Age.
- *Thou shall engage in self-talk and limiting statements that hasten decline.* It's supposed to be cute and funny, but it's not. It can be devastating. Remember that the subconscious listens to every thought you think and every word you say and will do its best to get or achieve what you spend most of your time focusing on.
- *Thou shall look forward to leaving the real world and moving to a retirement village where thou can safely practice thy religion with like-minded believers.* Retirement communities insulated from much of the real world will not help put old on hold. How can anyone hope to stay ageless and healthy when exposed to non-stop decline? Walled-in residents reinforce each other's infirmities, attitudes, beliefs and behaviors. Those unable or unwilling to venture out beyond the walls become victims of their static, controlled environment.

- *Thou shall abdicate responsibility for thy health and welfare to thy doctor and other experts who claim to know better than thee what's best for thou.* After all, it's a given that after age 65, thy brain doesn't function as well as it used to. Doctors know a lot but not one of them knows everything. As the expression goes, God helps those who help themselves. Regular reminders that because you are not as young as you used to be, that's the cause for everything that ails you, and it fuels your reliance on experts.
- *Thou shall start counting down to "D" or death day at age 60 if not sooner. Meaning thou shall first consider the number of years thou imagines thee has left before engaging in a long-range project.* That means, don't consider working on a degree or writing a book. Don't start the business you always dreamed of because you might die before you make your first million.
- *Thou shall take pride in referring to thyself as an "old geezer" or "old broad" and associate only with like-minded congregants for thee has found pleasure in the adage "misery loves company."* You have a choice. You can be an old broad or an old geezer or you can be a god or a goddess. The choice is yours, and which designation you choose will determine how others see you and relate to you. I guarantee, when the god or goddess mentality takes hold in your mind, you will stand taller, your thinking will be clearer and you will feel and look better physically.
- *Thou shall buy into the entitlement mentality and consider thyself a victim if indulgences, gifts and discounts are not forthcoming.* No, thou shall not. Righteous, upstanding

gods and goddesses don't ask for what they don't need or to what they are not entitled. Extending your hand for a handout compromises your regal stature.

- *Thou shall join seniors-only organizations and subscribe to seniors-only publications.* It's another manifestation of "misery loves company." Such publications, filled with ads for cemetery plots, hearing aids, dentures and seniors-only communities are comforting to peruse to those who sit and wait for the inevitable.
- *Thou shall not have a relationship with another adult significantly younger than thee unless thou are a male.* The rationale here is that much older males, even if cranky, crotchety and unattractive are entitled, because of their age, to have the affection of a sweet young thing. No one blinks an eye. If they have sired a child at a ripe old age all the better, in which case, they are regarded as a virile phenomenon and can go on talk shows and (wink-wink) show off or talk about the fruit of their erectile capacity. Case in point, eighty-something celebrity Tony Randall. After the birth of his children by his young wife, there he was on talk TV, looking great of course, and everyone understood the unspoken message: Tony is still a stud! (But let's not be cranky here. Bully for Tony!)
- *If thou are a woman over 50, thou certainly shall not have a relationship with a younger man* unless *thou are a celebrity.* It's difficult for an "ordinary woman" to have a relationship with a younger man in our judgmental society unless you are Mary Tyler Moore who is married to a man 18 years younger, or Tina Turner who is with a

man 16 years younger. The list of female celebrities who are with younger men include Joan Collins, Carol Burnett, Francesca Annis (this one is really sinful – she's 58, he's 39), Susan Sarandon, or Madonna. Obviously, this is one tenet of the Religion of Chronological Age that really irritates me. I definitely disapprove of an older woman having a relationship with a man under age 30 but once men and women are over 40, she should be able to have a relationship with whomever she chooses without suffering the stigma of "cradle robber". Gender enlightenment, anyone? But then, that's another book.

- *Thou shall make repeated references to chronological age, which gives credence to prevailing thought and conventional wisdom that says at any given age, thou should think and act in a manner befitting the social or cultural expectations for that age.* At age 40 you know how you are supposed to behave. It's your last chance to do fun and crazy things, like partying and drinking too much. May as well do it now because pretty soon, it's going to be all over! At age 50, if you are not thinking about retirement, there may be something wrong with you. If, on the other hand, you are taking tap dancing lessons, your sanity definitely is in doubt. At age 60, if you are thinking about going back to school, conventional wisdom says that's a waste of time. Social expectation can be a cruel master.

These and other existing articles of faith that our society buys into confirm we do indeed worship the numbers. We venerate chronological age, placing it on a high altar and we bow low before this destructive, controlling idol. This is one leap of faith we don't need. Run, brothers and sisters before it's too late! Redeem yourselves! Set yourself free from all the "must not do," "cannot do," "shall not do" cultural commandments that hold you back from becoming ageless!

Be a Birthday Party Pooper

Think about this: If you didn't know your chronological age, how would you live, think, and behave? Mind you, I'm not asking, "If you didn't know your age what age you would be?" as that question perpetuates the obsession with chronological age. If all you had to go on was past experience, your desire to realize unfulfilled dreams, and the condition of your health, finances, and personal obligations, what would you be doing? Without a constant reminder of how many years you may have left to live, how would your life be different? The point is, do not allow chronological age to dictate the terms and agenda for how you live your life. Ignore the numbers and all of the negative inferences attached to them. Live the way you want to live, and do what you want to do, instead of holding yourself back with excuses about being too old. As the Nike ads say, just do it!

As a child, I can't recall the number of times I heard my mother lament, "If only I were ten years younger . . ." or "If only I felt better . . ." She lived to 92, and as much as she accomplished, which was a good deal for a woman of her era, she forfeited many opportunities to fulfill her dreams because of her age or physical condition. In retrospect, her ailing condition was more often in her head than physical. People use all kinds of excuses to prevent success. If you are one of those "if only" kind of people admit it and ask, "Why do I shoot myself in the foot when opportunities come my way?" Decide how to stop this self-defeating thinking, particularly as it relates to your ability to put old on hold. If you can't figure out why these patterns keep repeating themselves, and you truly want to stop, it may help to work with a cognitive therapist. I suggest a cognitive therapist because they don't have you rehash your childhood to try to find what's wrong. They deal with what's happening now and what you can do to make things better, regardless of what happened in the past.

Don't allow awareness of your chronological age to limit your potential. Put less emphasis on birthday celebrations. (And boy, do I know that's a hard one to give up, especially if they involve family get-togethers.) Nevertheless, I suggest you give up birthday celebrations. At least try to wean yourself from them. If you think about it, birthday parties are kid stuff. You and your family celebrated your birthday on day one of your life; that was the most important birthday you will ever have. For those who belong to the Church of Chronological Age this annual event is a gloomy acknowledgment of the past and a tyrannical and unnecessary reminder of what little time may be left. I stress the words, "that *may* be left" because no one knows when that final moment will occur. That alone is depressing, but what's worse is when friends send a cute but hurtful reminder of your mortality, commonly known as a greeting card.

For example, how do you feel when you receive a card with a sentiment such as this: "Hey, Babe, you are finally 50! So what if you are over the hill! Take your arthritis medicine and boogie the night away if you can stay awake past 8 P.M." Sure, you giggle but you may not realize how it can destroy your self-image and accelerate your aging process. It's just one incident, but the effects are cumulative. A little bit here, a little bit from there, and the result is an insidious chipping away at your confidence. Remember, you may shrug off the silliness but your subconscious doesn't discern what's real and what is not. People you love and trust have told you that you are over the hill. Whether you consciously choose to believe it or not, your subconscious accepts the message. It sinks in, takes hold and influences the evolution of how you perceive yourself. This in turn affects your aging process.

Next to depressing greeting cards, there are the gifts. Perhaps friends throw a party and present you with tokens of love in the form of ExLax and a bottle of Geritol as a reminder you are slowing down in more ways than one. Then they lavish love on you with these supposedly supportive comments:

"You're really holding up well for your age, dear."

"You look a little stiff; is your arthritis bothering you, darling?"

"You took tired, sweetie. You're not overdoing it, are you?"

"Did you get your invitation to join AARP?"

"A new senior community is opening. Seems like a nice place to retire."

Talk about exasperation! I'm tempted to utter a nasty four-letter word, but I won't say it out of respect. Common expressions should not assault the ears and eyes of gods and goddesses.

Better than a Party: The Blast That Lasts All Year

Not to worry. There is a better way. Tell friends and family not to send birthday greeting cards because they will be unopened, marked return to sender and put back in the mailbox. And tell them don't bother to give "cutesy" gifts that are demeaning and undermine your efforts to put old on hold.

Sure, parties are fun, but you have something better going on. Let everyone know that instead of celebrating once a year, you have a put-old-on-hold agenda for the next twelve months. If anyone wants to participate, welcome him or her warmly. Plan to do at least one or maybe more activities each month that will help you put old on hold. Then do it! Here are twelve suggestions:

> Month No. 1: Cut out all greasy, expensive snack foods from your diet. Watch the weight melt away and your savings increase. Now that's something to celebrate! It's the gift that keeps on giving.
>
> Month No. 2: Enroll in an exercise class or invest in a treadmill and use it. Put it in front of your TV (so what if it clashes with your décor), and strengthen your cardiovascular system while even more weight falls off. Isn't that more exciting than a calorie-laden birthday party?

Month No. 3: Read a book by a nutrition guru and put into practice what makes sense to you. Then read another health-related book and another. Share what you learn with your unenlightened friends.

Month No. 4: Get a new hair style and color. Why wait another year to update your appearance? So what if you look better than your peers look? Maybe it will motivate dull or drab friends to get a new look going, too.

Month No. 5: Replace clothing that dates you. Donate discarded items to a tax-exempt organization and remember to declare it as a deduction on your income tax. You certainly can't take a deduction for a birthday party!

Month No. 6: Sign up for a computer class at your local college, or a community education program. Enroll in a voice or drama class. If there is a latent computer nerd or star-struck diva within you, now is the time to go for it! Don't advertise what you plan to do, just do it and then amaze everyone with your newfound knowledge and skills.

Month No. 7: Start laying the groundwork for the dream career or job you've always wanted. Network and talk to people who know the field you want to get into. Put your plan in writing, review it, refine it, and add to it every day. Start saving a predetermined amount of money every month to help fund your dream career. By the same time next year you will really have something to celebrate.

Month No. 8: Find more opportunities to interact with young people. Meet them in church activities, classes, community programs and at work. Volunteer to coach or supervise a youth program. Offer to teach what you know that you take for granted but will open up a new exciting world for them. Be aware that it's often difficult for young people to relate to older people. So be open and non judgmental, and they may share some thoughts that will wake up your brain cells. Celebrating their positive qualities will help you put old on hold.

Month No. 9: Do something your family, friends, social custom or tradition say you are not supposed to do at your age. If it's not illegal or immoral, just do it! If you must have a party, throw one to announce your intention to learn how to sail a boat, tap dance, ice skate, sky dive or become a brain surgeon. Make sure you intend to do it; this is not the time to be a wannabe.

Month No. 10: Change your TV habits. Be extremely selective and cut the number of hours you do watch the tube. Read or do something active to help you stay fit and vital. If you must watch TV, do it while you exercise. Have you ever walked or exercised during a birthday party? Well, perhaps dancing could be considered exercise!

Month No. 11: Volunteer at a local senior center or convalescent home. It's a perfect win-win. You do a good deed and get a bird's eye view of debilitating old age. It will motivate you to work your plan to put old on hold. Guaranteed.

Month No. 12: Review your accomplishments for the past months and start a new, better-than-ever plan for the next 12 months.

After you successfully complete your first year of putting old on hold, invite others to join in your monthly commitments. You will feel the power of healthy choices and know you are disconnecting from chronological age. Share your successes, and celebrate your program! Give them a copy of this book!

Gods and Goddesses Just Do It!

These rules matter only after you have first accepted and adopted the heart and soul of the three major concepts: Health, Retirement and Attitude. I'm assuming you have done that and now you are ready to tie all the pieces together. So, copy the list of rules from the Table of Contents and stick it on your bathroom mirror, refrigerator door or wherever you can frequently see it, read it and think about it. I guarantee that with your determination to put old on hold these rules will positively shape your evolution as an ageless god or goddess.

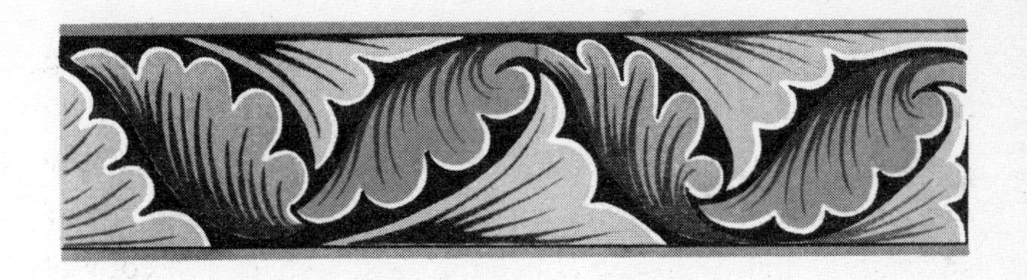

Mission Possible: Putting Old on Hold

I have an admission to make: It's lonely being an ageless goddess. I need you beside me on my ageless pedestal – there's plenty of room for you and others to prove that the damaging earth is flat attitude about aging is wrong and needs to be changed. I'm counting on you to become a role model and help others to become gods and goddesses. Will you do it? I'd sure appreciate it. To refresh you memory about what I've already said about what it takes, here are points I want you to remember.

- Love yourself; not in a narcissistic sense, but in recognition that you are a valuable human being with a valuable life. When you value what you have, in this case, your body and your life, you are less inclined to abuse it with alcohol, food, tobacco or neglect. Always hold your head high and keep your shoulders back. I don't want your tiara to become askew.

- Believe it's possible to put old on hold. That may seem difficult or impossible for many people, but I remind you of the time in history when the most respected scholars in the universe decreed the earth was flat and everyone believed. It was an irrefutable truth until someone sailed off into the horizon and did not fall into a black hole. I've sailed into the horizon of old age and I know what's beyond the horizon; it's a terrific second life for those who follow my program. The reality is that much of the decline associated with the aging process is nothing more than the result of a lifetime of abuse and neglect. That's why you must first value yourself. If you think about that deeply and often enough, you will come to understand how valuable you are, and will do what it takes to change your life forever.
- Visualize, and commit to attaining what you desire. Doors will open; you will make intuitive choices that propel you toward your goal. In my case, because I knew what I wanted to achieve, early on I began yoga exercises which have kept me flexible. I began to exercise with Jack LaLanne and that has helped me to stay in shape. I read books by nutrition pioneer Adele Davis. I devoured Prevention and Organic Gardening magazines when founder J.I. Rodale was in charge. I heeded the advice of Nobel Laureate Linus Pauling when he extolled the value of mega doses of Vitamin C. In other words, I intuitively did many things needed to put

old on hold. I continue to seek out ideas and information that promote healthy longevity.

The first three ideas above are necessary precursors for the rest of the points given below. You have to be ready and willing to change. If you value yourself, believe you can achieve your goal to put old on hold, and commit to your goal; then you are well prepared to accept and practice the following points.

- Health is primary. Without superior health, nothing else matters. Not money, sex, power, status or fame. But you can have it all when you have exceptional health. You can remain youthful, healthy and productive regardless of age. Believe this. Make a commitment to acquiring and maintaining your health. It's not enough to simply think it might be a good idea. Action makes it so. Commitment will require changes in your lifestyle. So welcome these necessary changes and know you are making the best decision for yourself, your family, and your future.
- Educate yourself about optimum diet and nutrition. Gradually phase out the deficient, debilitating, All-American diet and replace it with tasty, healthy fare. Remember, just because something is advertised as food doesn't mean it's good for you. Don't abuse your body with what you put into your mouth. You weren't born loving greasy fries and burgers and gooey sweets that make you sick and old. You are capable of making good

choices. You can learn to love anything that promotes good health. Eat less, and eat more high quality food. Learn about diet supplements, even if you eat a balanced diet. Ultimately you will save money as well as your health. Drink pure water, lots of it and you'll remain a juicy plum instead of becoming a dried-up prune.

- Find a traditionally trained physician who has developed expertise in anti-aging medicine and nutrition. This will go a long way to help you reach your goal to put old on hold. An anti-aging physician will do things a traditional one won't, such as regular blood tests that reveal more than you could possibly imagine, and necessary to know about if you want to mitigate the aging process. Blood tests today are so sophisticated in what they can discover and uncover; they are a true snapshot of what's going on in your body.
- Engage in rigorous mental management and mental discipline. No more "I must be getting old" or "I'm having a senior moment" comments. Establish an exercise program and discipline yourself to stick with it. You will do it if you have internalized that you are valuable and worthy and deserve to have a healthy long life.
- Monitor how you are changing over time. Work to keep youthful attributes. What are youthful attributes? Observe old people and note what it is about how they live, how they move, how they think that is old and resolve to avoid what bothers you. A couple of youthful attributes worth keeping are the ability to stand tall and

move with youthful agility. Decide what's important to you, and work relentlessly to get it.

- Observe behaviors of family members. We tend to emulate the thinking and behaviors of those nearest and dearest to us. Expressions such as "She's just like her mother," or "She's become just like Aunt Mary" tell it all! It's okay to become like your mother or other family members if they are exceptional role models.
- Train yourself to avoid the systematic countdown syndrome "I may have only X years to live" as an excuse for not having long-range plans. Stay future oriented while fully living in the moment.
- Goals fuel longevity and good health. Acknowledge the reality of death with appropriate legal preparation and other arrangements, then approach life and live with full commitment every day as if you will live forever. That's right, I said forever. Think positively.
- Think of traditional retirement as a degenerative disease; a fast track to decline, decrepitude, and an early demise. I urge you not to even consider retirement. If you retire from a career position and move on to some other productive and challenging livelihood, don't call it retirement. Think of it as your second life.
- Prioritize and maintain a structured daily schedule of essential activities such as exercise, eating properly and visualization to help you put old on hold. Follow this schedule regardless of what happens. Don't answer the phone, don't allow interruptions, and don't put up with your own silly excuses for putting it off just this one

time. Stay in control when the part of you that doesn't want you to succeed raises its ugly head. Thoughts such as "I don't think I'll bother today" must be immediately replaced with "Oh yes I will!"

- Include young people in your environment. Yes, they can sometimes be a nuisance but they are also a source of energizing joy. In their inexperience and immaturity, they are often exquisite teachers of curiosity, understanding, and disarming innocence. Adopt the best of their thinking and behaviors, especially their freshness of thought and, in return, demonstrate the best of your experience and maturity to help them grow into wise adults. The exchange or energy and vision between yourself and a younger person can provide hope, and motivation, and optimism for your respective futures.
- Avoid those seniors-only organizations and publications that subscribe to the Church of Chronological Age, giving an inescapable impression the end is near. Those subtle and not so subtle messages have a devastating effect on your subconscious and therefore on your conscious behavior. If you routinely read publications that carry advertisements for cemeteries, cremation, hearing aids, dentures, reverse mortgages and seniors-only housing, you might be tempted to sail off into the sunset. The seniors who read these publications, rely on them, appreciate them and most insidiously believe in them, aren't putting old on hold. They are putting their precious lives on hold.

- Instead of seniors-only publications, read books and materials that encourage growth, challenge, and productivity. Read what inspires, informs, and motivates you to grasp all of the opportunities available to you, in spite of and regardless of your age. Educate yourself to get the most out of your life every single day you are on this planet.
- Avoid being a proselytizer, disciple, or martyr of the Church of Chronological Age. To be sure you are not a follower or believer, periodically review the major tenets of this bogus belief system. Every time you review them you may gain new levels of enlightenment.
- Consciously and deliberately develop a pattern of positive self-talk. When someone asks how you are, always reply, "I'm wonderful" with enthusiasm even if you feel awful. Tell your tales of woe only to those paid to listen. Friends will always be happy to spend time with you if you avoid burdening them with your problems.
- Live in a spirit of constant gratitude for your many blessings. However many or few blessings you have, take stock of them, keep them in the forefront of your consciousness, and give thanks. Is your arthritis pain better today than yesterday? Be thankful. Verbalize it. Can you stretch a little farther today than yesterday? That's an improvement, so be appreciative. Acknowledging gifts, being aware of improvements in your life, and expressing gratitude for them (particularly when you are having a less than perfect day), releases a

flow of endorphins (happy hormones) in the brain, which in turn infuse you with a sense of well being. This joyful state lights up your eyes and face, doubling as a beauty treatment. It makes you more open and connected to others. Your positive attitude will allow more good things to happen. It works for me and I know it will work for you.

- Choose friends carefully. Avoid those who try to diminish your youthful vitality. Stay away from people who expect a lot but give nothing in return. Select friends who share their positive outlook and level of vibrancy so you can feed off each other's energy and be a source of support on the few occasions where it is needed.
- Seek out role models and copy their behaviors and emulate their attitudes. Always be on the lookout for attitudes and practices that foster growth and positive change. Be a role model for young people as well as your peers. Project an aura of vitality and inner peace that others notice (far more than you may think) and they will want to emulate.
- Work to maintain your inner vibrancy. It's a highly youthful characteristic. Let the world see the light radiating within you. Let your energy and vitality set you apart from the bitter old people whose sour expressions say it all. Consider the attractiveness of young people who project a glowing, animated awareness and interest in what's going on around them. Being other-oriented is a gift that comes with youth. As the years go by and we become more preoccupied and self-absorbed, this gift

diminishes but it can be restored. Choosing to cultivate an alert sincere interest in others will give you a more youthful appearance. It will make you feel better, too.

- If you don't already have one, develop a positive, uplifting, and outrageous sense of humor. Teach yourself to laugh at a problem you won't remember next week. Consciously and deliberately brush off most of life's small stuff irritations with a smile. Laughing heartily every day and wearing a smile, will keep you young and healthy. You will look better, feel better, and be better company, too.
- Defy convention if it holds you back from reaching your goal to put old on hold. Constantly be on the lookout for the many subtle ways conventional thinking may sabotage a youthful, vital productive future. If there is something you want to do but believe you shouldn't attempt at your age, just do it anyway. What is the worst that can happen? Even if it's a disaster, you'll have an amusing story to tell plus the satisfaction of knowing you gave it a good try.
- Revel in standing apart from the masses of aging, conforming lemming-like human beings heading toward the deep abyss of premature old age. Don't be afraid to march to the beat of your own drummer, and if there is someone you truly care about, try to gently lead them in your direction.
- Be a rebel and a leader. Delight in running ahead of the pack, showing the way to agelessness by your vital example. As you bypass the road to traditional old age,

reach out to others and encourage them to join you. Take them by the hand or under your wing and nurture them as they develop strength and conviction. Soon they will learn to soar agelessly on their own. Encouraging others to take charge of their lives is powerful beyond imagination. It has a boomerang effect. The more people you help to live agelessly, the longer you will stay vibrantly young and healthy yourself. This strategy works for me and will work for you, too.

The Opportunity of a Lifetime

Understand that putting old on hold is not merely about maintaining a more youthful appearance, although looking good as you age is one of the payoffs for taking care of yourself through the years. The real benefit of putting old on hold is maintaining your personal power. It's getting to age 60, 70, and beyond, feeling and functioning like a healthy 40 or 50-year-old. When you possess excellent mental and physical health, you can do just about anything you choose. You can go back to school, embark on a new career or a new business, or take up a new hobby. It's about being in charge of your life for as long as you choose. It is being able to revel in freedom and independence, and having choices and opportunities such as these:

- It's freedom from financial worry. When you are healthy, you can work and have a job that allows you to enjoy an abundant lifestyle instead of living at poverty level, dependent on paltry Social Security checks, or an equally inadequate person.

- It's freedom from fear of mental, physical or emotional abuse. You will be able to fend off well meaning friends and family whose objectives may not be the same as yours.
- It's freedom for yourself and your adult children by giving them the gift of not having to worry about crucial issues such as moving you into a long term care facility, moving in with the children, or having to assume financial responsibility.

No one can remain young forever but everyone can enjoy ageless qualities until the day they die. I am so eager for you to achieve agelessness that I'm going to ask you to do one thing for me before you finish this book. Right now, close your eyes and imagine yourself at age 60, 70, or beyond. See yourself physically strong, mentally sharp, and healthy. See yourself looking much younger than your years, full of youthful energy. Savor this picture so you'll remember it and hold it in your mind's eye. You're anticipating wonderful things to come and doing what you want to do because you are in prime, peak condition. Feel the power you have because you've consciously controlled your lifestyle choices. This visualization is the first step in your plan to put old on hold. Do this exercise tomorrow, the next day, and the next, until it becomes an automatic part of your daily routine. Each day, visualize your future self in ever sharper detail and you will *become* your vision. I guarantee it; you *will* put old on hold!

Your determination and action plan to put old on hold will help explode myths and misconceptions about aging and what constitutes old age. Your commitment to achieving healthy agelessness is a vital role in achieving positive change. Join the few, the mighty, and the determined ones who have made the decision to maximize their true potential. There are some readers who may simply put this book down and go on with their lives as always. My heart goes out to them. I have let you in on powerful information few people understand. You may not have realized it but reaching the end of this book marks a completely new beginning for you. I've done my best; the rest is up to you. Please write and tell me what you are doing, how you've used the information, and how it has changed you and your life. I'd really like to hear from you. My address is PO Box 937, Escondido, CA 92033-0937. My email is *PutOldonHold@aol.com*. Or visit my website at *PutOldonHold.com*.

Resources

To keep you from being immobilized with options, I'm providing you with a list of excellent resources so you can start gathering information. The number of resources and amount of information available today on health maintenance can be overwhelming. Feeling overwhelmed is the last thing you need if you are just beginning your mission to put old on hold. This resource list is what I have found helpful at this stage of my life. Over the years, I've sifted and sorted through tons of material and narrowed down what works best for me. Having said that, please don't stop with what you find here. You too will need to go through tons of information before you find what works for you. Let this be just the beginning of your quest. (Note: Phone numbers, addresses, and websites may be subject to change.)

Books

The Antioxidant Miracle, Lester Packer, Ph.D., w/Carol Colman, John Wiley & Sons, 1999. Essential Reading to understand the Free Radical Theory of aging.

Drug-Induced Nutrition Depletion Handbook, Ross Pelton, et al., Natural Health Resources, 1999. You must have a copy of this in your home!

Juicy Tomatoes, Plain Truths, Dumb Lies, and Sisterly Advice About Life After 50, Susan Swartz, New Harbinger Publications, 2000.

Grow Young with HGH, Ronald Klatz, w/Carol Kahn, Harper Perennial, 1997. If you have an interest in human growth hormone (HGH) this is the book to read.

Eat Right for Your Type, Peter J. D'Adamo, w/Catherine Whitney, G. P. Putnam's Sons, 1996.

Your Body's Many Cries For Water, F. Batmanghelidj, Global Health Solution, 1995. Buy it!

Cosmetic Surgery: Before, Between and After, Susan Gail, Melange Unlimited, 2000. Be prepared. Read it before you need it!

Retirement is Over-Rated, Donald R. Germann, M.D., Leathers Publishing Productions, 1998.

Brain Longevity, Dharma Singh Khalsa, M.D., w/Cameron Stauth, Warner Books, l997.

The Perricone Prescription, Nicholas Perricone, M.D. Harper Collins, 2002. Dietary simplicity and common sense. Plenty of medical expertise, recipes, and recommendations. Before and after photos show how diet can profoundly affect appearance of the skin. A must read.

How to Find Great Senior Housing, Phyllis Staff, Ph.D., TBIY Publications, 2002. This book is the most exhaustive, easy-to-understand resource for finding the best living accommodation for your loved one in need of long-term care.

Why is Everyone so Cranky?, C. Leslie Charles, Hyperion, 1999. Is there anyone who doesn't need an attitude adjustment from time to time? There aren't enough superlatives to describe this incredibly helpful book.

Stick to It!, C. Leslie Charles, Yes! Press, East Lansing, MI, 1995. This little gem will encourage and support your determination to put old on hold. A fast, easy and nourishing read!

Magazines

Life Extension
1881 North 26 Street, Suite 221
Wilton Manors, FL 33305
phone: 954-561-7909
e-mail: Lemagazine@lef.org
website: www.lef.org
Life Extension magazine is a must for serious anti-agers.

Let's Live
11050 Santa Monica Blvd.
Los Angeles, CA 90025
phone: 310-445-7500
e-mail: info@letslivemag.com
website: www.letsliveonline. com

Also, visit your health food store for free magazines. Don't discount their value just because they are free. They can be an invaluable source of information.

Newsletters

Dr. Julian Whitaker's Health & Healing
Phillips Health
7811 Montrose Road
Potomac, MD 20859
phone: 800-539-8219
website: www.drwhitaker.com

The Sinatra Health Report
Stephen Sinatra, M.D., F.A.C.C.
Phillips Health
7811 Montrose Road
Potomac, MD 20854
phone: 800-211-7643
website: www.drsinatra.com

The above two newsletters and websites are "musts." Yes, these two physicians sell vitamins and supplements as well as other health related products but the information they provide is exceptional.

Websites

www.putoldonhold.com
www.drsinatra.com
www.drwhitaker.com
www.womansage.com
www.minniepauz.com
www.susangail.com
www.reverseaging.org

Miscellaneous Information

Carol Maggio Facercise
6960 Eastgate Blvd.
Lebanon, TN 37090
phone: 615-449-8877

ACAM American College for Advancement in Medicine
23121 Verdugo Drive, Suite 204
Laguna Hills, CA 92653
phone: 949-583-7666,
800-532-3688
www.acam.org
Helpful for finding an an alternative or integrative physician

American Academy of Anti-Aging Medicine
phone: 773-528-4333

Directory of Innovative Doctors
Life Extension Foundation
phone: 800-544-4440

For comprehensive blood testing:
www.yourfuturehealth.com

Life Extension Foundation also offers blood tests. Check out their website <www.lef.org> for current information.

Newsletter

If you are interested in receiving Barbara Morris' email newsletter, please send an email to *PutOldonHold@aol.com*. Just write "Subscribe" in the subject line. The newsletter provides health and anti-aging information you probably won't find elsewhere. When you subscribe, please include a note about the kind of information you particularly want to see in the newsletter.

Barbara Morris on the Internet

Barbara's website:
www. PutOldonHold.com

Email:
Barbara@PutOldonHold.com

Index

AARP, 106–107
acid reflux, 72
Adderall, 49–50
adult children, 16, 120–121, 181
advertising:
  Baby Boomers targeted, 80–81
  Direct to Consumer (DTC), 29–31, 74–75
  example set by, 72–73
  for junk food, 48–49
age, 5–6
  chronological, 5–6, 159–164
  inner, 146–148
  revealing to others, 4–5, 137
  See also aging; specific topics
"age spots," 61
"ageless culture," 3–4
agelessness, 26–27
aging:
  decline associated with, 8–9, 83
  oldness, 3–4, 10–12
  premature, 6, 8, 103
  social expectations regarding, 11–12, 26, 33–36, 104, 159–163, 179
  (*See also* relationships)
  two models for, 3–4
  See also specific topics
AIDS (HIV), 62
alcohol, 8, 46, 171–172
  See also wine
alpha lipoic acid, 60–61
Alzheimer's disease, 36, 151–152
  iron and, 77
  polyphenols and, 61
American diet, 28, 40–43, 45–54, 80, 173
antacids, 71–73
antibiotics, 79–80
anticonvulsants, 57–58
antioxidants, 59–62
anxiety:
  about the future, 34–36
  and serotonin-deprivation, 56
  "small stuff," not sweating, 134
  See also specific topics
appearance, 5, 87, 138–141, 154–155, 168, 180
  cosmetic surgery, 141–144
  dental enhancement, 141–144
  facial expression, 137–138, 179
  posture, 123–124, 144–145, 174–175
arteries:
  blockage, 60–61
  folic acid for, 21
aspirations, *See* goals
asthma, 62
Attention Deficit Disorder (ADD), 49–50
attitude, 8, 12–14, 25–26, 111–114
  gratitude, spirit of, 177–178
  negativity, *See* negativity
  positive self-talk, 177

thoughts, power of, 145–149, 159
See also specific topics

B vitamins, 46, 56–57, 62
Baby Boomers:
adult children, *See* adult children
advertising targeted to, 80–81
fears held by, 34–36
Batmanghelidj, F., M.D., 70–71
Bennett, Tony, 129–130
bioflavonoids, 62
birth-control pills, 56–57
birthdays, 164–167
blessings, appreciation of, 177–178
blood pressure, *See* high blood pressure
blood tests, *See* CBC/Chemistry profile
body, human, 54
caring for, *See* health
See also specific topics
boredom, retirement and, *See* retirement
braces (dental enhancement), 141–144
Brain Longevity (Khalsa), 35
bran, 50, 63
bread:
Alvarado Street Bakery, 63
white, 52
whole-grain, 50–51

C, vitamin, 56, 60–62, 172
smoking and, 22
caffeinated beverages, 69–70
calcium, 62
imbalance, correcting, 77
calories, *See under* diet
cancer, 24
antioxidants and, 62
and hormone imbalance, 77
iron and, 77
polyphenols and, 61
vitamin E and, 61
See also specific topics and conditions
cataracts, 62
CBC/Chemistry profile, 76–78, 135
centenarians, 3, 113–114
cereal, 28, 50–53
Channing, Carol, 127
children:
adult, *See* adult children
and Attention Deficit Disorder, 49–50
See also young people
China, 28
chiropractic therapy, 55
chlorine, 66
cholesterol levels, 10, 17–19, 53, 57
chondroitin, 64
clothes, *See* appearance
coenzyme Q10, 57, 60–61
coffee, 69–70
cognitive therapy, 165
congestive heart failure, 57
Conquest of Happiness, The (Russell), 100
convention, *See under* aging: cultural expectations regarding
cosmetic surgery, 141–144
Cosmetic Surgery: Before, Between and After (Gail), 141

Davis, Adele, 172
death:
destructive attitudes regarding, 161, 176
final expenses, 107
preparations for, appropriate, 109
subconscious perceptions regarding, 12 (*See also* subconscious)
dehydration, *See* water consumption
dementia, 36
dental enhancement, 141–144
dependence, avoiding, *See* independence
depression, 56, 83, 94–95
and hormone imbalance, 77
treatments for, 73–74
Dexedrine, 49–50
diabetes, 10, 24, 57
causes of (type II), 52–53
and hormone imbalance, 77
vitamin C and, 62
zinc and, 57

diet, 9–10, 25
  American, *See under* American diet
  and food abuse, *See* food abuse
  and obesity, *See* obesity
  restricted calorie, 10, 27–28
  and supplements, nutritional, 55
  See also supplements, nutritional; weight loss
difficult people:
  dealing with, 111, 135–136
  entitlement mentality, *See under* entitlement mentality
  reasons for behavior, 100–103, 135
  See also relationships
Dilantin, 57–58
Direct to Consumer (DTC) advertising, 29–31
diuretics, 57, 69
doctors, 17–18, 22–24, 26
  alternative/anti-aging, 26, 39–40, 43, 174
  over ninety, 117
  partnering with, 26, 39–40
dreams, *See* goals
dress, *See* appearance
Drug-Induced Nutrient Depletion Handbook (Pelton), 58
drugs, *See* medications
dyspepsia, 72

E, vitamin, 60–61
eating, *See* diet; food
education:
  about your health, *See under* health: educating yourself
  learning, lifelong, 152–154, 168
  reading, 126, 177
  school, returning to, 108, 163
  See also mental sharpness
eggs, 51
employment, *See* work
energy, 25, 77, 178–179
entitlement mentality, 99, 118–121, 155–157, 161–162
exercise, 26, 121–125, 157–158, 174–175
  skills, evaluating, 131–132
  weight-bearing, 11
eyes
  cataracts, preventing, 62
  macular degeneration, preventing, 61

face:
  exercise for, 125
  expression, 136–138, 179
  See also appearance
face lift, *See* cosmetic surgery
family:
  adult children, *See* adult children
  behaviors of, observing, 11, 175
  inherited conditions, *See* genetics
  overprotective, 120–121
  pressures by, *See* aging: cultural expectations regarding
  See also relationships
fasting, 43–44
fat, body weight, *See* diet; weight control
fat, dietary, *See* diet
fiber, dietary, 63
finances, *See* money
financial planning, 107–109, 168
flaxseed, 28
fluoride, 66–67
folic acid, 21, 56, 62
food, 8
  abuse, 40–43, 45–54, 80, 171–173
  processed, 45–54
  See also diet
Free Radical Theory of aging, 10, 59
friends, 6
  choosing, 126, 178
  observation of, 11
  See also relationships; specific topics
future:
financial and legal planning, 107–109, 168
goals for, *See* goals
  See also specific topics

Gail, Susan, 141
gastrointestinal problems, *See* stomach problems
genetics, 13–14, 24, 27, 73
Germann, Dr. Donald R., 109–110
gingko biloba, 60
glucosamine, 64
glucose, high serum, 77
goals, 96, 110, 131–133, 168, 175
  planning for future, 107–109, 168
  social pressure, overcoming, 143
  visualizing, 145–149, 181
  See also growth, personal
gradualism, 11, 111–112
gratitude, spirit of, 177–178
"greens" supplement, 63–64
Grow Young with HGH (Klatz), 43
growth, personal, 12, 104
goals, *See* goals; learning, lifelong
gum disease, 60–61

Happiness, The Conquest of (Russell), 100
Harvey, Paul, 115–116
health, 13–28, 173
  and chronological age, 5–6
  educating yourself, 37–39, 168, 173
  fears regarding, 34–36
  problems, *See* health problems, below
  taking responsibility for, 17–19, 28, 34, 36, 81, 161
  See also diet; specific topics
health care system, 29–37
  doctor, choosing, 39–40
  HMOs, 29–31
  See also doctors
health problems:
  dealing with, 137–138
  declining health, 8–9
  See also specific conditions and topics
heart attack, cutting risk of, 61
heart disease, 24
  gum disease and, 60–61
  vitamin E and, 61
heart medications, 57
heartburn, 72
  water and, 70–71
herbs, 55
  See also supplements, nutritional
heredity, *See* genetics
high blood pressure, 10, 24, 53
  and CoQ10, 57
  folic acid for, 21
high serum glucose, 77
Hittleman, Richard, 125
HIV/AIDS, 62
HMOs, 29–31
Holliday, Cliff, 116
homeopathy, 55
human growth hormone (HGH), 43–44
humor, 134, 179

income loss, 83–84
independence, 14, 26, 98, 119–121, 157, 179–180
Indole-3-carbinol, 63
insurance, 107
  health care system, *See* health care system
integrative physicians, *See under* doctors: alternative/anti-aging
iron, 77

jobs, *See* work
junk food, *See* American diet

Khalsa, Dharma Singh, M.D., 35
kidneys, 78–79
kindness, 135–136
Klatz, Dr. Ronald, 43

LaLanne, Jack, 128–129, 172
learning, lifelong, 152–154, 168
  See also education; mental sharpness
leisure time, 100–104
Life Extension magazine, 130–131
lifestyle, 27–28, 34
  anti-aging, 9–10
  heredity vs., *See* genetics
  See also specific topics
limitation thinking, 114, 117
  See also negativity

liver, 78–79
  and drug side-effects, 18–19
love of self, 25, 171–172
low-calorie diet, *See under* diet: restricted calorie
Lynette, Sadie, 114–115

macular degeneration, preventing, 61
Maggio, Carol, 125
magnesium, 56, 62
maintenance, need for, 112–113
managed care (HMOs), 29–31
medications, 17–19, 29–33, 72–81
  advertising of, 29–31
  cost of, *See* health care system
  food abuse and, 80
  multiple, use of, 75–76
  necessary, 72, 75–76
  and nutritional supplements, 56–58
  prevention vs., 23–34
  sampling program, 31–32
  and side effects, 56–58, 74–75
  See also health care system
medicine:
alternative, 55
  (*See also under* doctors: alternative/anti-aging)
  See also doctors; health care system; medications
memory, 35–36, 151–152
  gingko biloba for, 60
  See also mental sharpness
men:
  and appearance, 155
  See also specific topics
menopause, treatment for, 78
mental attitude, *See* attitude
mental sharpness, 25, 125–126, 157
  retirement and, 12, 14
  (*See also* retirement)
  and skills, evaluating, 131–132
  supplements for, 60, 157
  work and, 87–88
  See also education; learning; memory
mid-life crisis, 15–16
migraine headaches, 63
money, 15–16, 34, 173, 180–181
  and health care, *See* health care system
  work vs. retirement, 83–84, 88–92
  See also financial planning
MSM (methylsulfonylmethane), 64
multiple sclerosis, 63

negativity, 8, 148–149
  "limitation thinking," 114, 117
negative self-talk, 26, 149–163
  See also attitude
nicotine gum, 20
nursing homes, 85
  See also under retirement: housing
nutrition, *See* diet
nutritional supplements, *See* supplements, nutritional
nuts, 28

oatmeal, 28, 50–51
obesity, 48, 53
  and hormone imbalance, 77
"old age," *See* age; aging; specific topics
oral contraceptives, 56–57
osteoarthritis, 63
osteopathic physicians, 40
osteoporosis, 10–11, 57
  preventing, 123
overweight, *See* diet; obesity

Parkinson's disease, 63
  iron and, 77
patience, showing, 135–136
Pauling, Linus, 56, 172
peer pressure, *See under* aging: social expectations regarding; relationships
Pelton, Ross, et al., 58
physicians, *See* doctors
planning:
  goals, *See* goals
  See also specific topics
plastic (cosmetic) surgery, 141–144
polyphenols, 61

positive attitude:
positive self-talk, 177
  See also attitude; specific topics
possessions, 15
  See also money
posture, 123–124, 144–145, 174–175
  See also appearance; exercise
poverty, *See under* retirement: and income loss
power, personal, 15, 173, 180
premature aging, *See under* aging: premature
prescription drugs, *See* medications
Prevention magazine, 58–59, 172
processed food, *See under* food: processed
prostate cancer, preventing, 61
psillium, 63
public assistance, 16–17

reading, 126, 177
  health-related, *See under* health: educating yourself
relationships, 14–15, 26
  group mentality, 99, 117, 160
  helping others, 14, 87–88, 130–131
  new, 16
  positive role models, *See* role models
  with young people, *See under* young people: relationships with
  See also aging: cultural expectations regarding; specific relationships
relatives, *See* family; genetics; relationships
rest, 93–94
restricted calorie theory of aging, 10
  See also under diet
retirement, 12–14, 83–110, 159–160, 175
  housing (retirement communities), 99–100, 106–107, 117, 160
  and income loss, 83–84, 90–92, 97, 101
  lifestyle, 86, 98–100
  productive, 86–87, 97, 103
  seamless living vs., *See* seamless living
  and self-esteem, 95–96
  as traumatic break, 104
  work vs., *See* work
Retirement is Over-Rated (Germann), 109–110
Ritalin, 49–50
Rodale, J. I., 58–59, 172
role models, 114–117, 126–131, 178
routine, daily:
the retirement lifestyle, *See* retirement
  value of setting, 175–176
Rowe, Dr. John, 27
Russell, Bertrand, 100

salt, 69
SAM-e (S-adenosylmethionine), 63
schedule, daily:
  the retirement lifestyle, *See* retirement
  value of setting, 175–176
school, *See* education
seamless living, 104, 109
self-esteem:
  accomplishment and, 153
  work vs. retirement and, *See* retirement; work
  See also specific topics
self-love/respect, 25, 156, 171–172
self-reliance, *See* independence
self-talk:
  negative, *See under* negativity: negative self-talk
  positive, 177
  (*See also* attitude; goals)
"senior citizens":
  group-mentality relationships, *See under* relationships: group mentality
  See also specific topics
senior communities, *See under* retirement: housing
"senior culture," 3–4
"senior moments," 26, 35–36, 151–152
seniors-only organizations, 176
serotonin, 56
sex, 15, 173
Sinatra, Dr. Stephen *(Sinatra Health Report)*, 43

skin care:
  "age spots," 61
  water and, 25, 70
slant board, use of, 124–125
"small stuff," not sweating, 134
smoking, 8, 19–22, 171–172
  vitamin C and, 62
social expectation, *See* aging: cultural expectations regarding
Social Security, 16, 31, 91, 101, 108, 110, 181
soy, 28, 62
stomach problems, 47, 53, 71–73
  See also specific conditions
stress, *See* anxiety; specific topics
stroke, 60–61
subconscious, the, 12, 89–90, 148, 151, 160, 166
  See also attitude; thoughts
sugar, *See* diet; specific topics
supplements, nutritional, 54–64
  anti-aging, 58–62
  drinking and, 46
  for mental sharpness, 60, 157
  organic, 58–59
  smoking and, 21
  See also specific topics and conditions

teeth:
  dental enhancement, 141–144
  gum disease, *See* gum disease
television, 169
thankfulness, spirit of, 177–178
therapy, cognitive, 165
thoughts:
  negative, *See* negativity
  power of, 145–149, 159
  subconscious, *See* subconscious, the
  See also attitude; visualization
tobacco, *See* smoking
tolerance, showing, 135–136

vacations, 93–94
viruses, preventing, 61
visualization, 25, 148, 172, 175, 181
  See also goals; subconscious, the
vitality, *See* energy
vitamins, *See* nutritional supplements; specific vitamins
volunteer work, 97–98, 169

walking, *See* exercise; posture
Wallace, Mike, 127–128
Walters, Barbara, 127
wardrobe, *See* appearance
water consumption, 25, 28, 44–45, 64–71, 174
  chlorine and, 66
  fluoride and, 66–67
  steam-distilled water, 65–67
water pills, *See* diuretics
wealth, *See* money
weight-bearing exercises:
  for osteoporosis, 11
  See also exercise
weight control:
water and, 68–69
  See also diet
welfare, *See* public assistance
Wellbutrin, 20
whey, 62
Wiggins, James Russell, 114
will, drafting, 109
wine:
  polyphenols in, 61
  See also alcohol
women:
  and society's expectations, 162–163
  See also specific topics
work, 3, 5, 116
  benefits of, 87–89, 92–93, 97–98, 103, 180–181
  and retirement, *See* retirement
worry, *See* anxiety; specific topics
wounds, healing, 62

yoga, 123, 125, 172
young people, 11, 15–16, 174–175, 178–179
  relationships with, 88, 98, 117–118, 128, 162, 168–169, 176

Your Body's Many Cries for Water (Batmanghelidj), 70–71
youth, characteristics of:
keeping and regaining, 111–113, 131–132
See also specific topics
zinc, 56
diabetes and, 57
Zyban, 20

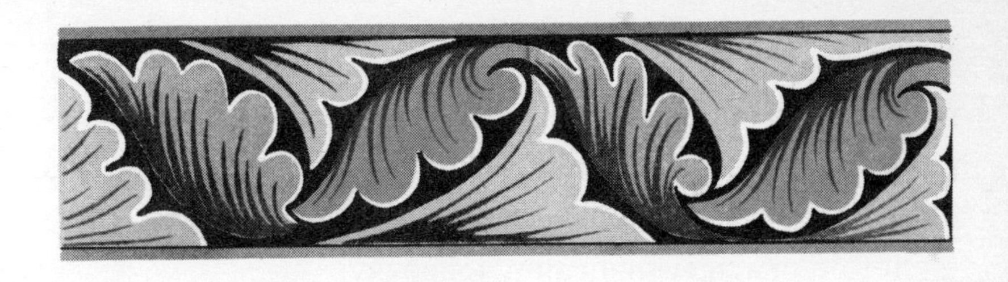

Barbara Morris' Personal Anti-Aging Program

Most adults, regardless of age, would like to be healthy or would like to begin a prevention and maintenance program, but they don't know what to do or where to start. In this book, I have urged you to educate yourself about what it takes to develop a healthy, anti-aging lifestyle, and I have provided resources to nudge you in the right direction.

The Put Old On Hold™ Program

However, I believe there is a need for more specific direction regarding dietary supplement recommendations, so I asked experts at Longevity Labs to put together a unique vitamin supplement system specifically designed for those interested in embarking on a strong, anti-aging program. I wanted superior formulations I could offer at a reasonable price.

The program had to include an abundance of anti-aging anti-oxidants as well as essential ingredients not typically found in ordinary "over-the-counter" formulations. I specifically wanted to help people taking a certain type of anti-cholesterol medication. Let me explain why I am so concerned about this particular type of medication, especially for those interested in achieving healthy longevity.

Currently, the most widely used drugs to control cholesterol are known as "statin" drugs. While they effectively control cholesterol they also deplete an important substance called CoQ10, which is vital for a healthy heart and prevention of muscle pain and deterioration so I wanted to include a significant amount of CoQ10.

Aside from medication-induced vitamin depletions (cholesterol lowering drugs are but one example; there are many, many more), if you are not taking vitamin supplements, or if you are taking a drugstore "daily multiple" that provides just the government-approved minimum daily requirement, chances are you are not getting enough of what you need, not only to keep your body running well from day to day, but to build up your immune system to protect against future health assaults. Your goal should be to take supplements with enough muscle to keep you running in peak condition, now and in the future. My Put Old on Hold™ supplement program meets that requirement.

Nutritional Bankruptcy

Statistics say 90 percent of money spent on food is spent on processed food that in large measure is nutritionally deficient. As a pharmacist working in a supermarket pharmacy, I see what's in shopping carts: Bags and bags of greasy chips;

boxes of expensive nutritionally deficient "breakfast cereals"; prepared dinners loaded with chemicals you can't pronounce and which your liver was never intended to detoxify; loaves of white bread as soft as cotton and about as nutritionally useless; jugs of mostly colored sweetened water advertised as healthy drinks; cases of expensive, nutritionally worthless sodas. Research shows that phosphoric acid in colas keeps calcium from being absorbed and that women who drink more than three 12-ouce servings of cola a day have 2.3% to 5.1% lower bone mineral density in the hip than women who consume less than one serving of cola a day. Osteoporosis is not a disease of "old age," it's due in large part to a damaging diet. The amount of money wasted on nutritionally deficient food choices is astronomical, and the long-term effect on health is disastrous. Love and protect yourself by taking care with what you put into your mouth.

I also see a lot of wine, whiskey, and vodka in shopping carts. Alcohol is dehydrating and many people do not drink enough water to begin with. Your body needs lots of water to function optimally. Theoretically, every glass of wine or beer you consume should be followed by a glass of water to compensate for the alcohol-induced dehydration. If you drink vodka or whiskey, it is even harder on your body, and requires replenishment of even more water.

The other thing about alcohol is that it robs the body of essential vitamins and nutrients, especially B vitamins. Alcohol is a nutritional thief. You submit your body to a felonious assault when you drink alcohol and do not at least partially compensate with water and vitamin supplementation.

Even if you do not abuse alcohol and eat unhealthy semi-foods, chances are you are consuming more than is good for you. Not only that, even a 'healthy" diet is often nutritionally deficient. Considering how fresh food is often grown, stored, shipped, and treated with preservatives and chemicals to delay deterioration, counting on diet alone to provide what your body needs is not wise.

The Good News

Here is the good news: with superior dietary supplements, you can atone for some dietary and lifestyle transgressions and the questionable value of some "fresh" food. I am often asked, "Which vitamins should I be taking?" I could rattle off a laundry list that might confuse or frustrate you. Instead, I will just recommend my Put Old on Hold™ Program. For a little over a dollar a day, you will give yourself a great gift that will really pay off now and long term. You can check out the ingredients before your buy. If you imagine you cannot afford the modest investment in your health, think about how much money you might throw away on some of the above mentioned nutritionally useless edibles that masquerade as "food."

Love and value yourself enough to get started on the road to superior health and youthful longevity. Try my Put Old on Hold™ Program by visiting:

http://www.reverseaging.org

If you don't take care of yourself, who will? Please don't wait. You deserve the best loving care you can give yourself.

The earlier in life you begin, the greater will be the payoff when you are 60, 70 and beyond. I'm doing it; you can do it too.

About the Author

Barbara Morris is a graduate of Rutgers University College of Pharmacy and works full time as a retail pharmacist.

As a child whose early years were profoundly influenced by an often-ailing mother, Barbara decided early on that she would never grow old and dependent. This was no fleeting childhood fantasy. Barbara quickly realized that staying young, vital and healthy was more of a possibility than anyone imagined.

As a young woman she became convinced that signs of "old age" associated with the aging process were not just the result of heredity, but also, the result of lifestyle choices that could be deliberate and controlled.

Now in her seventies with physical and mental characteristics and abilities of someone many years younger, it is clear that Barbara's beliefs about how to achieve agelessness were right on target and are paying off even better than she had hoped.

In entering what Barbara calls her Second Life, she is dedicated to helping others realize their dream of retaining characteristics of youth; a goal she insists is absolutely achievable. She contends that anyone willing to take the steps she has taken can replicate and perhaps even exceed her success.

Barbara enjoys reading, writing, working crossword puzzles, and fantasizes about becoming a professional ice skater when she grows up. Her husband Marty, a former college professor now into his second career as a pharmacist, has maintained his love for research and, as a result, Barbara insists he is the smartest man in the world. As expected, traditional retirement is not part of their life plan.

Their many blessings include a daughter, two grandchildren, and a home in Southern California, the closest place to paradise on earth, except when the earth shakes.